Laura!
This book is perfect
for a (secret) newlyw
Banish the plain un
enter a world of roman
beneath-the-clothes excitement
Yaay!,
Suzanne Kelley

UNDERNEATH IT ALL

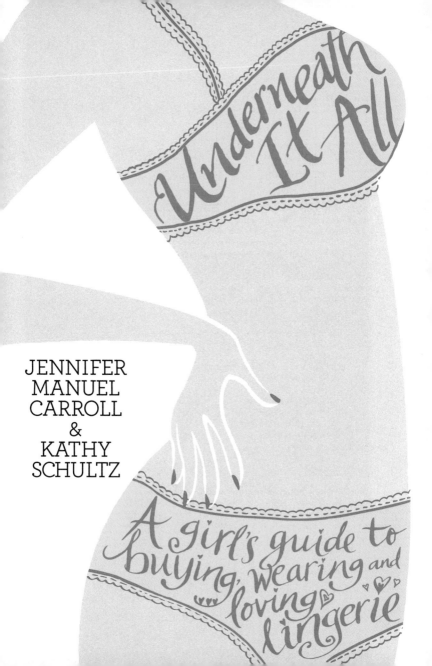

Underneath It All

JENNIFER
MANUEL
CARROLL
&
KATHY
SCHULTZ

A girl's guide to buying, wearing and loving lingerie

HARLEQUIN™

Underneath It All

ISBN-13: 978-0-373-89205-1
ISBN-10: 0-373-89205-5

Library of Congress
Cataloging-in-Publication Data
Carroll, Jennifer Manuel.
    Underneath it all:
    a girl's guide to buying, wearing, and loving lingerie /
    Jennifer Manuel Carroll and Kathy Schultz.
        p. cm.
        Includes index.
    ISBN 978-0-373-89205-1 (pbk.)
    1. Lingerie. I. Schultz, Kathy II. Title.
    TT670.C37   2009
    646.4'204--dc22

    2008051431

www.eHarlequin.com

Printed in U.S.A.

Acknowledgments

There are many people who have touched my world of lingerie and helped make this book a reality. Thank you to my husband, Ryan, for encouraging me to spend more time and money on my underwear than on a steak dinner at El Gaucho. *Muchas gracias* to my friends Kim Destro and Elif Eroglu, who inspired me, over margaritas in Belltown, to write this book. Big thanks to my reformed-hippie mama, whose bra boycott fueled my passion for all things bra related. Merci beaucoup to my coauthor, Kathy Schultz, for making this a fun and adventurous collaboration involving lots of beer, French fries and laughs. Much appreciation goes to Jennifer Unter, my stellar agent, who had faith in this project; to all at RLR Associates, who have been a great support through the process; to Leela Corman, our sassy illustrator; and, of course, to the wonderful team at Harlequin, Deborah Brody and Sarah Pelz, without whom this book wouldn't exist. Lastly, a heartfelt thank-you to all my wonderful customers, family members and friends, who teach me lessons in life, love and lingerie on a daily basis.

♥ Jen

First, a sincere debt of gratitude to my best friend and longtime husband, Dean, for his support during this project, and his acute appreciation for nice lingerie. To Lisa Wogan, who has been a wonderful friend and cherished colleague through my whole writing career, your encouragement and editorial eye have been invaluable. Thanks to our agents: Tara Mark, for getting the ball rolling, and Jennifer Unter, for keeping it in the ballpark and running with it. My appreciation goes to editors Sarah Pelz and Deborah Brody for their editing expertise. Kudos to Robin Kilrain, a longtime writing buddy and crackerjack copy editor, and to Leela Corman, illustrator of cool girls. To all the women who contributed their personal lingerie stories, thank you. We wish had room for all the tales, juicy as they were.

And lastly, but mostly, I want to acknowledge my coauthor and friend, Jennifer Carroll, for bringing me in on the project. It was a most delightful experience and so much fun to work with a lingerie expert extraordinaire who is not only creative and hardworking, but also kick-in-the-panties funny.

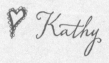 Kathy

Contents

LOVE YOUR UNDERWEAR, LOVE YOURSELF

Lingerie is one of life's pleasures. Shouldn't it be something you love? If you've been reaching into your underwear drawer every day for the same old style of panties, putting yourself into an uncomfortable bra or thinking you don't look good in lingerie, we have news. Whether you have minimal cleavage, an ample booty, or an apple- or pear-shaped body, there is beautiful lingerie out there for you!

The state of your underthings can actually change your state of mind. How many of us have picked a pair of panties we liked because we were feeling good that day? Or rummaged around our drawers for a pair we disliked because we woke up feeling down in the dumps? Instead, imagine putting on sexy French lingerie underneath your business suit and feeling excited and empowered, or putting on a flirty bra beneath a T-shirt and feeling feminine and confident.

Lingerie should be chosen with as much care and thought as you choose your makeup. You need the perfect foundation before you start making yourself beautiful with blush, mascara, eyeliner. Lingerie is the same way. A foundation that fits well means more-flattering clothing. Your undergarments can make or break your look: smooth T-shirt bras make that tight white T look like a million bucks; the right panties under tight pants will have people doing a double take (and not because you have visible panty lines); and shapewear can smooth out lumps and bumps in that clingy cocktail dress. We could go on and on. And we will.

Just like fashion, lingerie is a form of self-expression. When you pair a corset top with a pencil skirt, or switch out plain hosiery with nude fishnets, you're showing your sense of style and making a statement.

Intimate apparel also mimics fashion by following color and cultural trends. You probably wouldn't wear the same style of shoes for years on end, so it's logical that your tastes and choices in lingerie also evolve and change through the decades.

In our twenties, we primarily dress in lingerie for our men. In our thirties, we learn to wear and appreciate lingerie for ourselves. In our forties, we can either run into a rut or learn about new styles and how to wear them. In our fifties and beyond, we may feel basics are the way to go, or we may choose to splurge on luxury lingerie as a treat. As decades go by, we discover that wearing lingerie transcends putting on a bra that fits. It's more about embracing our femininity, enjoying our bodies and cherishing ourselves.

No matter your age, with the help of this book you will learn how to enjoy lingerie in everyday wear, transforming the concept of "underwear" into lingerie you love. Both lingerie virgins and veterans will gain insight into their own lingerie styles and receive practical tips on how to confidently and correctly wear intimate apparel. From bras to hosiery, we'll sort it all out and expose what these underpinnings are all about. We'll suggest brands for every shape and budget. Brides-to-be will benefit from our tips on wedding and honeymoon lingerie. We'll give you a little history lesson, chronicling important lingerie dates, events and milestones. We will even give you seduction scenarios—in the event your imagination runs less than wild.

All you'll need to do is invest a bit of time determining your style and needs. We'll hold your hand and walk you through it. Trust us, it will be well worth the investment. Think you're alone in the process? Au contraire! We have included personal stories from women of all ages and with all different body types about their escapades and experiences with lingerie.

So let's get going and find out what's *really* underneath it all. But before we do, here's a little about us and how we came to write this book.

Jen: My Love Affair with Lingerie

When I grew up in the 1980s, lingerie was as much a part of fashion as it was part of pop culture. If you remember the lace anklet socks and pumps, you know what I'm talking about. From a young age I was significantly influenced by the fusion of lingerie and everyday wear.

In junior high I worshipped Madonna: I sported white, fingerless lace gloves and layered multiple lace shirts over my training bra. I even donned a fake above-the-lip mole one year at camp. (It was eyeliner; shhh, don't tell anyone.) By the time I was in high school, it seemed like a natural progression to shop at Victoria's Secret and Frederick's of Hollywood at the local mall.

As a high school sophomore I wore fishnets under my cutoff jeans. I dressed in a garter belt with thigh highs under skirts at sixteen. At nineteen I frequented a local reggae venue in northern California, where I wore a burgundy velvet bra and not much else. The doorman never carded me. I felt feminine and powerful—and I still can't believe my mom let me out of the house. By the time I finished college, lingerie was a beloved part of my wardrobe, something that held memories of hot summer concerts and adventurous young love.

On a trip to France in 2001, my boyfriend—now husband—and I found ourselves in a little shop on the Champs-Élysées called Lise Charmel. He bought me a sheer, black demi bra and knickers set with delicate, red floral embroidery. It was breathtaking. Even on sale, it cost more than one hundred and fifty dollars. I couldn't believe he splurged like that. Later, when I put the set on for the first time, I felt completely transformed. My man gasped when I walked out of our hotel bathroom.

I couldn't stop smiling. It was then I discovered the true power of lingerie—and also developed my champagne taste for underwear.

My love of lingerie drove me to open my own shop in Seattle a year later. The journey has been educational and never dull. Helping women with their underthings is a very intimate experience, and it requires a lot of trust on each customer's part. I assist women in finding their actual bra size, which celebrates and enhances their breasts: "Yes, my love, you *are* a 34C, not a 36A. Enjoy!" I also specialize in picking out the perfect cut and style of lingerie for each woman's body type. It has been extremely gratifying to help women express themselves through their lingerie, while encouraging them to have fun along the way.

The idea for this book came about over cocktails with some girlfriends. Following a couple of margaritas, the conversation turned to how to wear lingerie for a man. After an entertaining and educational discussion—and more than a few hoots and hollers—my friends said, "You should write a book!" I considered my conversations over the years with customers and their questions about lingerie, from practical to naughty, and I realized women could use a lingerie book about what to wear and how to wear it.

As for my personal relationship with lingerie, these days my routine has simplified. As a wife, mother and business owner, I don't see nightlife very often and don't always have time to pamper myself. My intimate apparel is one thing I don't skimp on, so I always have a little luxury in my daily life. I feel alluring when I put on a beautiful nightgown before bed, and I feel put together because my bra and panties match and are flattering. But most of all, I adore the realization that I am taking care of myself by loving the first thing I put on my body: my underwear. Frankly, I deserve this little bit of luxury—all women do.

Thus, my love affair with lingerie continues. This book is dedicated to all you lovely ladies who are ready for a new adventure. Enjoy!

Kathy: My Life in Lingerie

My earliest memories of falling in love with lingerie were in a St. Louis auto repair garage in the 1960s. My grandfather owned it and my father worked there with him. (I know it sounds bad, but stay with me here.) When I was a child, Mom would stop at the shop and my siblings and I would pile out of the car and say hi to Dad and Grandpa. We loved going there. Grandpa had a pop machine with a secret hand crank. We'd open the door and help ourselves to sodas, either chocolate or Vess cream. Grandpa gave us pennies for the peanut machine. We'd punch the green buttons on the circa-1940s adding machine, run up the incline on the wheel alignment rack and receive "rides" on the air jack from my dad. Standing on the hose, Dad would flip the air jack switch and up we'd go a couple feet. It was all great fun.

But one of my favorite activities was sneaking peeks at the pinup girl calendar behind the desk. The calendars were New Year's gifts from auto parts suppliers and the Snap-on tool company. I loved looking at the Vargas Girls, sexy watercolor and airbrushed paintings by Alberto Vargas from the 1940s. Lithe and well-endowed women with red-painted nails appeared in scanty lingerie, black stockings, tap pants, see-through nighties, diaphanous peignoir sets and mules. They were so exotic! I couldn't wait until Grandpa turned the calendar on the first of the month to see a new ensemble. I dreamed of the day I would be grown-up enough to wear these "outfits."

Fast-forward a few years to my first underwire bra in high school. I read they were an important invention to keep breasts from sagging. No one wore them then, and my best friend teased me mercilessly and called me Wire Woman. I also discovered colored panties in wild prints and—gasp!—black. I felt sexy in my sheer, shimmery nude bra in the 1970s. It was perfect under my body-hugging tops paired with bell-bottoms and platforms.

In the 1980s I discovered teddies and garter belts. What fun! My first teddies came in dusty rose and teal. I stepped outside the box and bought a red garter belt. I splurged on a merry widow. I scanned Frederick's of Hollywood catalogs for fishnet stockings. I bought matching bra and panty sets along with lots of colored lingerie and black, lacy underthings. My underwear drawer was filling up with naughty delights.

Despite my adventurousness, I could have used some guidance. I almost always wore the wrong bra size. I was close, but no banana, buying too big a band size and too small a cup size. In the late 1980s I finally got a fitting and figured it out. As the years went by, my taste for nicer lingerie grew, but my confusion about where to invest my hard-earned cash did as well. I bought impulsively, randomly and, often, unwisely.

That is, until I met Jennifer in 2003 and she helped me refine my taste. I've always liked classic, simple cuts without a lot of bells and whistles, sexy pieces and sophisticated black. Jennifer helped me build a lingerie wardrobe that is functional, flirty and flattering. She became a friend as well as my expert consultant. Both our friendship and my lingerie wardrobe continue to grow.

It's never too late to educate yourself and build a lingerie wardrobe that covers the bases with practical pieces and sensational ones you love—all you have to do is turn the page to get started!

UNDERNEATH IT ALL

*If God wanted us
to be naked, why did he
invent sexy lingerie?*

- SHANNEN DOHERTY

CHAPTER 1

Lingerie

A BRIEF HISTORY, FROM TOPS TO BOTTOMS

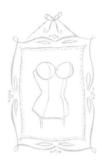

Lingerie has evolved in the last one hundred and fifty years, much to our collective relief. Imagine a world without breast-enhancing bras, an endless number of panty styles to choose from or that pair of lifesaving, figure-flattering SPANX in your drawer. Back in the day, options were limited. In fact, certain intimate pieces did not even exist. Before panties were invented at the turn of the twentieth century, you wore…nothing! (Going commando is nothing new.) The brassiere has progressed from little more than two hankies sewed together to a woman's inalienable right to have the best-fitting bra. Ladies, we are living in the golden age of lingerie.

The progression of what lies beneath has been historically influenced by many factors. These include need, function, social mores, economics, politics, fashion and beauty trends. What's more, an idealized concept of what constitutes a perfect figure has constantly changed and evolved, prompting women to alter their God-given shapes. Before we begin our whirlwind tour of the history of lingerie, we would like to discuss an area of anatomy that has been given a great deal of scrutiny, generates billions in revenue and grabs more attention than an exposed thong: the breasts.

The Rise and Fall and Rise of Breasts

Women's breasts have forever been at the mercy of fashion and beauty trendsetters, big business and society's mores. Throughout history, groups such as these have dictated what constitutes an ideal pair of breasts, be they flat, round, pointy, big or small. It's as if the breasts we were born with weren't good enough. Apparently, even the economy is a driving factor in their size. Lest you think that being well-endowed means being well-endowed financially, it's been said that flat chests are an indicator of periods of wealth. The trend toward smaller, flatter breasts, both in the 1920s and in the 1960s through the 1970s, occurred simultaneously with a healthy economy. In the future, we're just hoping for a healthy attitude toward breast size and shape, no matter if the economy is booming or going bust.

LATE 1800s TO 1920s

Breasts were not recognized as separate entities during the late 1800s. Breast improvers mushed things together into a "monobosom." From the early 1900s through the 1920s, many bra bodices flattened the chest into one matronly mass. The flapper styles of the 1920s turned the female silhouette into a boyish figure, with the approximate shape of a Hershey's chocolate bar. Breast-flattening contraptions were a girl's best friend.

1930s TO 1950s

Divide and conquer was the theme of the 1930s, when the bra as we know it showed up on the scene, lifting and separating. Pointy, uptilted breasts were in vogue during the 1940s. Models and advertisers show busty women leaning back, torpedo-breasts reaching for the heavens (a nod toward air travel and the future space program?). In the 1950s, voluptuous bodies took center stage. Marilyn Monroe, Gina Lollobrigida, Elizabeth Taylor...need we say more? Everyone on-screen looked ripe and luscious in their 34DD bras.

1960s TO 1970s

Chests flattened out again in the mid-1960s with Twiggy's arrival. There was little need for that 32AA model to restrain the girls. Bras took a nosedive. It was also an era of sexual and social freedom. This translated into freedom from the constraints of a bra, a trend that carried through the 1970s. Breasts were relieved of their bras, which were symbolically burned in bonfires. If worn, the trend was toward sporting glossy bras with see-through cups.

1980s TO 2000s

In the 1980s, breasts again became a focal point, with the return of erotic lingerie. Bras started to get gussied up. By the 1990s, we were bursting out of our bras as breast augmentation became as commonplace as blond highlights. As for the twenty-first century? Options are many: embrace your small pert breasts or your lusciously large rack. Enhance them or reduce them—the choice is now yours.

Baby Got Back

Though the focus on women's backsides has not been as great historically as that on breasts, big butts are gaining popularity. We cite favorite celebs such as J. Lo, Beyoncé and tennis star Serena Williams for callipygian glutei maximi. Following are some memorable moments in panties and padding throughout the ages.

MID- TO LATE 1800s

Before women were celebrated for their well-endowed posteriors, there was the bustle. With its inception around the 1860s, the bustle gave women the illusion of a wasp waist. Typically an apparatus attached to, and worn underneath the back side of a dress, it was originally designed so fabric draped downward. Eventually it developed a life of its own and, in the 1880s, rose to the occasion by elevating the rear, creating a shelflike appearance. One aesthetic purpose of the contraption was to balance the bosom and buttocks, forming the ideal figure of the late nineteenth century.

As for what lay underneath, women ran around commando during this period. Drawers were nonexistent. When they did make the scene, the open-crotch construction was considered hygienic. The design was convenient in the ladies room and for certain other (ahem) activities.

1920s

The fanny went as flat as an old tire, to complement the deflated chest of pencil-straight flapper girls. After a couple decades of debate on open- versus closed-crotch underwear, the case was sewed shut. Ventless panties won.

LATE 1940s TO EARLY 1950s

The 1930s paid little attention to the rear view, but in the 1940s the hourglass figure demanded a little more padding to balance the bosom. After taking a backseat to the breasts for so long, the bottom rose to the forefront in the 1950s. Pinups like the curvaceous Bettie Page and formfitting dresses à la Kim Novak made the posterior a focal point once again.

All girls wore tighty whities in the 1950s, under their poodle skirts and preppy pleated school skirts. Black may be in-your-face erotic, but in retrospect, there was something wildly sexy about women clad in white underpants and pointy-cupped bras.

True Lingerie Story:

Look like Liz

When my mother was engaged in the 1950s, she had a lingerie shower. Years later, when my sister and I were in our twenties, we discovered Mom's stash of slips. They were unopened, neatly folded in those thin boxes that lingerie used to come in. There had to be a dozen of them, and they were beautifully made with pleats, darts and lace. There were all colors: red, petal-pink, black and one with a beige lace top and black skirt. We always wore them around the house when it was hot. They make you look so sexy in that *Cat on a Hot Tin Roof* kind of way.

—*Maureen G.*, 34A

1960s–1970s

As body fat dropped à la Twiggy, so did the size of women's behinds. In the 1960s and 1970s, no one wanted a big butt. Slim was in. Panties shrunk in size and rise, the better to wear under all those miniskirts and low-slung hip-hugger jeans. (Nevertheless, girls with voluptuous booties were celebrated in the 1978 song by Queen, "Fat Bottomed Girls.") As for fashion, colored panties in wild prints mirrored the psychedelic styles of these decades.

1980s

By the late 1980s, the thong had crept into the underwear drawers of women nationwide. But it was still a runner-up to the high-cut Brazilian brief, which showed lots of thigh.

1990s

We see London, we see France, we see *everyone's* underpants. Thongs suggestively peeked out, or brazenly exposed themselves, from under women's low-riding jeans. Barely there underwear, such as the thong and G-string, became increasingly popular. The rear got into gear with workout videos such as *The Original Buns of Steel.*

2000s

The G-string becomes one of the fastest-selling types of underwear styles among women. Big bottoms take hold as buttock implants and enhancements gain popularity. We, however, would opt for padded boyshorts, such as those from Huit's Just A Kiss Magic Pulp collection, or a low-rise option, such as BubbleBuns from Bubbles Bodywear.

Great Moments in Lingerie through the Ages

MEET THE BRASSIER (OR A BRA IS BORN):
1800s–1919

- Corsets are the body-shapers du jour. They're blamed for a myriad of health issues and cited for physical and social constraints.

- 1876: Féréol Dedieu invents the garter belt.

- Early 1900s: First pairs of women's underwear appear— and they're crotchless!

- 1907: The word *brassier* appears in print in *Vogue*.

- 1912: The term is added to *The Oxford English Dictionary*.

- 1913: New York socialite Mary Phelps Jacob constructs a "brassier" from two handkerchiefs and pink ribbon. She sells the patent to Warner Brothers Corset Company for $1,500.

FLAPPERS AND FISHNETS:
1920s

- Breast flatteners are the fad to accommodate the popular boyish form.

- Flappers show off their legs in hosiery! Tan tones mimic the skin. Fishnets and stockings in gold and silver make first appearances.

- Late 1920s: Crotches close on panties.

ONE SIZE DOESN'T FIT ALL:
1930s

- Elasticized girdles are the preferred figure-control device.

- 1934: Betty Boop's garter is censored.

- 1935: Cup sizes for bras are developed. Warner's letters the cups A through D.

- 1939: Vivien Leigh's eighteen-inch waist in *Gone with the Wind* brings attention to wasp waists.

SILVER-SCREEN GLAMOUR:
1940s

- Glamour is the new standard: negligees and dressing gowns are common on the big screen.

- Howard Hughes uses airplane technology to build a better bra for Jane Russell in *The Outlaw*. She hates it.

- 1946: Frederick goes to Hollywood and reveals barely there black underthings to the lingerie-starved public. Movie stars frequent his shop.

TIME FOR THE HOURGLASS:
1950s

- Seamless stockings arrive!

- Curvy women rule. Women like Lana Turner, Sophia Loren and Ava Gardner dominate the silver screen.

- Women can buy bras from $1.97 to $4.90.

- 1955: Marilyn Monroe's tighty whities are exposed in *The Seven Year Itch*.

- 1958: Liz Taylor sizzles wearing a slip in *Cat on a Hot Tin Roof*.

SLIM IS IN:
1960s

- Lingerie goes minimalist and becomes more utilitarian and unisex.

- 1962: The miniskirt is hot paired with patterned hose, pantyhose and tights.

- 1966: Twiggy's straight-figured popularity takes the sexy curves out of lingerie.

- 1967: Mrs. Robinson (Anne Bancroft) seduces Ben Braddock (Dustin Hoffman) by revealing her sophisticated leopard-print lingerie in *The Graduate*. It's the antithesis to sweet white cotton bra and panty sets popular in the day.

SETTING THE GIRLS FREE:
1970s

- Bra burning is symbolic of social freedom. Women let it all hang out.

- The punk movement takes torn fishnets out of the trash and puts bustiers, garter belts and stockings on the street.

- 1977: Runners Hinda Miller and Lisa Lindahl design the first jog bra: the prototype is two jockstraps sewed together.

UNDERWEAR AS OUTERWEAR:
1980s

- The Madonna phenomenon takes effect and lingerie is widely worn as outerwear.

- 1986: Stay-up thigh highs displace the garter belt.

- Late 1980s: The thong makes its way into most women's pants.

- 1988: In the movie *Working Girl*, Melanie Griffith vacuums the house in her skimpy panties and demi-cup bra.

THE BIGGER THE BETTER:
1990s

- Thongs and G-strings become increasingly popular in the Western world, peeking out brazenly from everyone's low-riding jeans.

- Viewers worldwide tune in to watch Pamela Lee (then Anderson) flaunt her orbital breasts on *Baywatch*. Breast augmentation gains universal and public acceptance.

- 1990: Madonna struts her stuff in a Jean Paul Gaultier–designed corset during her Blonde Ambition Tour. The flamboyant contraption featured überpointy conical-shaped cups.

- 1994: The WonderBra is introduced in the United States. The now-famous bra was designed to create maximum and dramatic cleavage.

FIT AND FABULOUS:
2000s

- Shapewear gains market share: SPANX becomes a household name after Sara Blakely launches her company that sells footless tights that discreetly control jiggle.

- Bras with price tags of one hundred dollars and more become commonplace.

- 2001: Millions of eyes are glued to the tube to watch the first televised Victoria's Secret Fashion Show, with stacked models parading around in the latest provocative lingerie styles.

- 2004: Super Bowl XXXVIII halftime show controversy featuring Janet Jackson's "wardrobe malfunction." Americans are outraged when her right breast and star-shaped pastie are exposed during a choreographed dance with Justin Timberlake.

- 2005: Oprah's "Bra Intervention" educates millions of women about their ill-fitting bras. She urges all women to be properly fit.

You should
spend your money
on some nice lingerie.
Big wool cotton pants,
that just doesn't work.
You have to feel sexy.

- HEIDI KLUM

CHAPTER 2

Your Lingerie Style

FROM SIMPLE TO SEDUCTIVE

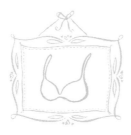

One of the greatest creative pleasures we enjoy as women is expressing ourselves through clothing. We can be wild fashionistas indulging in the latest trends, dress up in hot and sexy dresses or get comfy in jeans and a T-shirt. Picking what goes under our clothes is no different! Depending on our mood or style, we choose lingerie that makes us feel sweet, playful, sensual or practical. Some of us know absolutely what we love and what we hate. Some of us need a little help clarifying our style. And most of us need help putting it all together.

Find Your Style

The following quiz will guide you toward lingerie styles that best fit your personality and lifestyle. You may fall into more than one category or find yourself gravitating toward more than one style. That's great! It means you're open to more options. Once you find your style(s), read through the section(s) for some helpful tips on how you can take your lingerie wardrobe to the next level.

LINGERIE STYLE QUIZ
CIRCLE THE ANSWER THAT BEST FITS YOU.

1. When I try on clothing, I:
   - A. do knee bends to test for stretch/comfort.
   - B. check the fit and if the price is right, bingo!
   - C. imagine where I would wear my new purchase.
   - D. look at my butt in the mirror.
   - E. make sure it reveals my natural assets.

2. I typically buy lingerie:
   - A. at random.
   - B. at a department store.
   - C. at a mall store.
   - D. at a boutique.
   - E. anywhere, including a sex shop.

3. My favorite bra:
   - A. is comfortable.
   - B. works well under clothes.
   - C. is cute or frilly.
   - D. has a matching panty.
   - E. is sexy.

4. My handbag is:
   - A. a backpack or messenger bag.
   - B. basic leather.
   - C. multicolored.
   - D. coordinated with what I'm wearing.
   - E. the latest It bag.

5. My favorite sport is:

   A. running or biking.

   B. going to the gym.

   C. walking.

   D. Yoga or Pilates.

   E. bedroom antics.

6. My favorite shoes are:

   A. trainers or athletic shoes.

   B. black flats.

   C. a bright color.

   D. knee-high boots.

   E. high heels.

7. My favorite party
   refreshment is:

   A. a beer.

   B. wine.

   C. anything blended.

   D. a Cosmo or martini.

   E. straight-up anything.

8. My favorite kind of
   shopping is for:

   A. sports gear.

   B. food and beverages.

   C. home and garden.

   D. shoes and clothing.

   E. accessories.

9. My favorite perfume is:

   A. none.

   B. citrusy.

   C. floral.

   D. spicy.

   E. musk.

10. If I have a free evening I:

    A. go for a run.

    B. read a good book.

    C. call my friends.

    D. go to the theater.

    E. go dancing.

11. My favorite piece
    of lingerie is a:

    A. sports bra.

    B. panty.

    C. nightgown or chemise.

    D. bra.

    E. corset.

12. While on a date,
    I prefer to:

    A. do something active.

    B. stay in.

    C. double-date.

    D. have a deep conversation.

    E. make out.

13. My favorite panties are:

    A. boyshorts.
    B. cotton.
    C. bikinis.
    D. lacy.
    E. thongs.

14. My favorite parties are:

    A. Super Bowl
       Sunday parties.
    B. office parties.
    C. picnics.
    D. dinner parties.
    E. cocktail parties.

15. For pajamas I prefer:

    A. my boyfriend's shirt.
    B. a tank and pant set.
    C. something with a print.
    D. a chemise.
    E. to sleep in the buff.

16. My type of man is:

    A. athletic.
    B. handy.
    C. romantic.
    D. intelligent.
    E. successful.

17. Regarding hosiery, I:

    A. never wear hose.
    B. go for anything control top.
    C. love tights.
    D. always wear hose.
    E. love fishnets.

18. A robe:

    A. is not something I wear.
    B. should be warm and cozy.
    C. should have a
       pretty print.
    D. should be silky and sexy.
    E. should barely cover me.

19. When I entertain I:

    A. order pizza.
    B. have a potluck.
    C. spend weeks planning
       a menu.
    D. have it catered.
    E. make sure I have
       plenty of booze.

20. My favorite magazine is:

    A. *Shape*.
    B. *Real Simple*.
    C. *Marie Claire*.
    D. *Vanity Fair*.
    E. *Vogue*.

21. My idea of perfect transportation is:

   A. a Vespa or bike.
   B. the bus.
   C. a convertible.
   D. a European car.
   E. a sports car.

22. My idea of a perfect vacation is:

   A. an adventure trip to Costa Rica.
   B. at an all-inclusive resort in Mexico.
   C. a road trip.
   D. a trip to Paris.
   E. at a private island retreat.

23. My favorite bar is:

   A. a local sports bar.
   B. a restaurant bar.
   C. a karaoke- or live-music bar.
   D. a trendy lounge.
   E. a club with dancing.

Now count the number of marked answers in each column:

A Total: _____

B Total: _____

C Total: _____

D Total: _____

E Total: _____

Results: _____

Your highest score corresponds to your predominant lingerie style.

A: SPORTY

B: PRACTICAL

C: ROMANTIC/SWEET

D: SOPHISTICATED/CHIC

E: SEXY SEDUCTRESS

All about Your Style

Of course, we are all complex creatures and can't be defined by a single category. But the following descriptions will help you choose intimate apparel that fits your personality and lifestyle. Look them all over; they may give you ideas of other styles you want to try on for size. Your Lingerie Style might include one or more of the following:

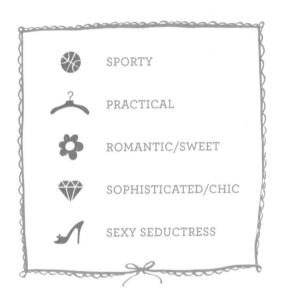

SPORTY

PRACTICAL

ROMANTIC/SWEET

SOPHISTICATED/CHIC

SEXY SEDUCTRESS

Throughout the book, these style icons will cue you to which pieces fit your personal style. Shopping just got much easier!

SPORTY

There are many underwear options out there for you Sporty girls, beyond jog bras. Your lingerie should be sleek and streamlined. And it should be made from material such as microfiber or Lycra, or a soft nylon mesh for comfort. Recommendations for you gals who want to "sport" lingerie while still keeping your athletic sensibility include the following:

- Sassy, soft bras comfortable enough to sleep in but also designed for support and daily wear.

- Comfy boyshorts that won't migrate during the daily routine.

- Simple thongs that will obliterate panty lines.

- Playful prints: stripes or tie-dye, floral or geometric pieces to keep things lively.

- Coordinated pajama sets in cheery colors or fun cotton camisole and short sets for sleeping.

BRANDS YOU WILL LIKE:
- Calvin Klein
- Gap
- DKNY
- OnGossamer

Tips & Tricks: Unless you are playing a sport, you should not be wearing a sports bra! They do nothing but restrict the movement of your breasts, pressing them into a boob omelet—not a tasty look.

Getting Started: Go out and buy a supportive bra that is so comfortable you forget you're wearing it.

A Note on Cotton

A true Sporty girl knows that cotton retains moisture. Just look at your running or cycling socks; they're not cotton. Though you might like cotton for your bras and panties because it's a natural fiber and you can wash and dry it with no worries, it's not the best choice for your underwear. Cotton bunches, stretches out of shape and holds sweat. If you must have this fabric, buy it blended with Lycra or another stretch fiber.

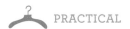 PRACTICAL

Who says practical has to be boring? You can be pragmatic and still wear exciting underwear! Pick items that are functional and fit properly but that also make you feel good. Invest in your underwear; it's the first thing that touches your skin. You deserve undergarments that make you look great and feel special. Here are some suggestions:

- A black T-shirt bra and matching black bikini. Simple and sexy—who knew?
- Camisoles with matching bottoms for sleep and daily wear under clothes.
- Cute print panties that have nude in the pattern to match your nude T-shirt bra.
- A thin cotton or modal robe in a soft, muted color to throw over anything.
- A shelf-bra tank with attractive lounge-style pants. Goodbye "boy beater" tank and sweatpants!

BRANDS YOU WILL LIKE:
- Chantelle
- Le Mystère
- Wacoal
- Gap
- Victoria's Secret

Tips & Tricks: Practical and stylish: If you have a black T-shirt bra, when it's time to stock up on panties, buy a bunch of black basic bottoms— thongs, bikinis or whatever. You will have a matching set every day without even trying!

Getting Started: Go to your favorite clothing store, visit their sleepwear section and buy a coordinated sleep set today. Stores such as Gap have loungewear sections with stylish separates that feel like a second skin.

❀ ROMANTIC/SWEET

You are a charming girl and it's reflected in your undergarments. Romantic girls are comfortable with coordinating, but not necessarily matching, sets. This will give you infinitely more shopping freedom! You like to freshen up your lingerie wardrobe, buying something new for each season. Look for these items:

- Flouncy, fun babydolls with floral or patterned motifs that celebrate your feminine side.
- Bras with bows, ribbons, interesting details and artsy straps to show off.
- Bottoms with ruffles, details and charm.
- Prints. Gingham and paisley and dots! Oh, my!

BRANDS YOU WILL LIKE:
- Betsey Johnson
- Elle Macpherson Intimates
- Felina Lingerie
- P.J. Salvage

Tips & Tricks: Be creative. If you find a killer deal on a cute camisole or bra (perhaps nobody bought the orange, purple or neon-green set), try to match it with a fun pair of panties. This will ensure you wear the item, and you will feel smashing in a (semi) matching set.

Getting Started: Go through your lingerie drawer and pick an item that you have been saving for a special occasion. Wear it today!

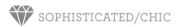 SOPHISTICATED/CHIC

You, lovely lady, need to wear things that make you feel beautiful. Nothing is off-limits for you, with the exception of "adult store" lingerie—and anything cheap or not luxurious. Some elegant recommendations include:

- Bra and panty sets that match perfectly.
- Lace in all colors and patterns.
- Designer prints, logo prints and colors.
- Chemises and gowns, to sleep in.
- Silk or satin pajamas.
- Long dressing gown or kimono-style robes, to wrap yourself in morning or night.
- High heels. Very high.

BRANDS YOU WILL LIKE:

- Aubade
- Cosabella
- Dolce & Gabbana
- La Perla
- Lise Charmel
- Simone Pérèle

Tips & Tricks: Always buy at least two pairs of panties to match each bra purchase. You may wear your bra two days before washing it, but never your panties.

Getting Started: Hang all your sleepwear on padded hangers in your closet. This way you can fill the "holes" in your lingerie wardrobe. What are you missing? Buy one new piece.

SEXY SEDUCTRESS

For you ladies, lingerie may be the most important part of your wardrobe. It's certainly something you lust for. As a Sexy Seductress, you have more than likely acquired several of these key pieces already. Keep your drawers stocked with:

- A silk nightgown and robe set, which will ensure you always have appropriate sleepwear when company is over....

- A silk camisole and tap pants set, for sultry summer nights.

- A corset or bustier, for those amorous moods.

- A pair of fishnets, thigh highs and stockings.

- A garter belt, of course!

BRANDS YOU WILL LIKE:
- Agent Provocateur
- Cotton Club
- La Perla
- Shirley of Hollywood

Tips & Tricks: Don't feel compelled to restrict your corset to the boudoir. Wear it out, over a skirt or jeans! You are a hot property, both inside and outside of the bedroom.

Getting Started: Because you truly love your undergarments, be kind to them. Refresh your bra and panty drawer today by washing all of your intimate apparel with a fresh-scented lingerie or hosiery detergent. Don't be afraid to launder your favorite delicate pieces; it's important to remove body oils from your fine silks and laces.

True Lingerie Story:

Everyday Indulgence

One summer I moved into a sublet with limited space and put most of my things in storage. I decided to package up my ugly underwear and only take the nice pairs. For a month I wore nice lingerie every day. Whether I went for a run or ran errands, I wore lacy or silky panties, and it made me feel fantastic. I realized I didn't have to save pretty lingerie, because I should feel special every day!

—Mara H., 32C

Brevity is the soul of lingerie.

- DOROTHY PARKER

CHAPTER 3

Lingerie 101

A LEXICON OF LINGERIE

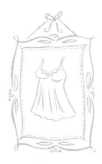

Intimate apparel has a vernacular all its own. *Demi, balconette chemise, tanga, low rise*—these are just a few of the terms frequently used in the world of lingerie. If you're baffled by the nomenclature of underthings and their specific purpose, you're not alone. This chapter is designed to give you a foundation about foundations and demystify what lies beneath. Here we provide concise definitions within the lexicon of lingerie and describe form and function. Following is a guide to each intimate piece, from the bras you wear every day to the garter belts you don for special ensembles.

Bras

T-SHIRT BRA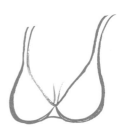

When you see a girl in a tight shirt and her breasts look smooth and perfectly round, she is probably wearing a T-shirt bra. This is an incredibly popular style for a reason: it is multifunctional and works under almost everything. It is a contoured-cup, underwire bra that has enough fiberfill to shape your breasts perfectly, regardless of shape or size. Those of you who see this bra as a piece of armor or think it is "padded" because of the fill, reconsider. Its structure is designed to make it remarkably supportive, not intended to add volume. It also serves as a great equalizer. If one breast is bigger than the other, a T-shirt bra is the solution because the cups will discreetly hide any discrepancy. Want to wear a tight white shirt without fear of a cold draft causing a scene? T-shirt bra to the rescue! Don it and dim those headlights.

CONTOUR BRA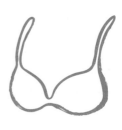

Are you looking for shapely, curvy breasts? (If not, you live on another planet.) The contour bra holds its shape with or without your breasts in it. Slip it on and voilà! Instant perfection. These bras come in every variety: demi, push-up, T-shirt and more. They are particularly

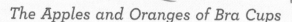

The Apples and Oranges of Bra Cups

A note on contour- versus molded-cup bras: While these terms are sometimes used interchangeably, they are, in fact, built with very different technologies. A contour bra has fiberfill and holds its shape with or without your wearing it. A molded-cup is created through a heat process that shapes the fabric over a breast mold so that the bra is seamless and breast shaped. The fit is trickier on molded bras, as the silhouette is fixed. If your breasts are augmented or not very full on top, this may not be your first choice.

helpful to those with breasts of different sizes or shapes, as the bra holds up its end of the bargain even if you fall a bit short. Wear it under anything and everything.

CONVERTIBLE/STRAPLESS BRA

A convertible is so versatile that it does everything but the dishes! It can be worn as a strapless, traditional two-strap, single-strap or halter bra. Most convertibles are shaped in a bandeau style (very Carrie Bradshaw in *Sex and the City*). You can also find them in plunge styles, with or without padding. Some strapless bras come without straps, period. But most come with two detachable straps to utilize as you please.

Strapless Suspense

It may seem impossible to find a strapless that actually supports your breasts while not compelling you to tug upward on your bra all day or night. When purchasing this style, consider the following:

1. Look for silicone around the band, which keeps the band from slipping down your back.

2. Choose a tight-fitting band that does not have to be on the tightest set of hooks to stay up.

3. Test the bra before purchasing, by putting your shirt on over it and walking around the shop a bit; if it slips now, it will most definitely slip later.

If you are over a C cup and don't trust any amount of silicone to hold you up, invest in a strapless bustier, which offers far more support. You can find details on the bustier in the "Special Items" section in this chapter.

PUSH-UP

Hallelujah! Praise this bra. It does exactly what it professes to do: pushes 'em up. This is the quintessential post-childbearing bra, for when breasts have lost some volume and need a little extra

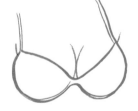

oomph. Most loved by A and B cup ladies, it's also adored by busty gals who need a little lift. The push-up bra typically plunges in the middle, with virtually no wire in between the breasts. It comes up higher on the sides and grabs your breast tissue, pushing it to the middle. This style is available in padded and unpadded varieties.

DEMI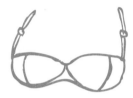

Sexy, sexy. Also called a half-cup, the demi is a bra with vertical seams and a very low bustline. The seaming creates a nice round look. It is a good style for most breast shapes and sizes, with the exception of those women who have a lot of upper-breast tissue that might spill over the cup. A demi looks great under low-cut shirts with scoop or square necks. It is an extremely popular gift for men to buy.

BALCONETTE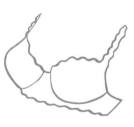

Stand up and be noticed! This sexy bra elevates breasts. The alluring yet practical style works well for most shapes. It often has a diagonally seamed bustline that offers a little more coverage than a demi bra, though some offer less coverage, depending on the brand. The underwires reach around and between breasts in a U shape. Horizontal or diagonal seams in a traditional balconette create a natural shape; vertical seams in a demi-balconette create a rounder silhouette. You can wear this bra under just about anything where seams don't matter.

Special Bras for Special Dresses

Clueless as to what to wear under that backless gown or halter-style cocktail dress? Join the club. Our tips for special occasion dresses will save you from a fashion meltdown before your big event:

HALTER

Choose a convertible bra that transforms into a halter or choose to go strapless. If the dress has a plunging back, you can buy a waist belt that turns your halter into a very low-back version that straps around your waist. If you need to go without straps and don't feel comfortable in a strapless bra, choose a bustier without straps.

STRAPLESS

Select a strapless bustier or bra. If the dress has a low-cut back, look for a long-line low-back bustier. Small-breasted women may consider having cups sewn into the dress or going sans bra.

SILK OR VERY THIN MATERIAL THAT SHOWS EVERYTHING

Buy a smooth, internally boned bustier; we like Le Mystère and Felina. Also wear control-top pantyhose or a support short pulled over the bottom seam of the bustier to erase any lines. For dresses with straps, you can invest in a one-piece bodysuit that creates a smooth silhouette. If you are in terrific shape, you might want to go commando and opt for a microfiber bra or discreet nipple covers to protect against air-conditioned venues.

CORSET-STYLE

Under this type of dress, everything works. Romantic lingerie sets or ruffles and lace—anything goes! If your dress has internal support or boning, you can consider going without a bra entirely. Sometimes the least complicated answer is the best one.

UNDERWIRE

These are beloved by the well-endowed and minimalists alike. A traditional underwire bra has soft fabric, smooth or lacy, and an underwire. The cups may be seamed, or molded and seam free for a smooth look under clothes. They typically have 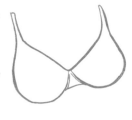 more coverage than a demi or balconette, and they are fabulously supportive and comfortable, with zero padding or fill.

RACERBACK

If you are constantly adjusting your straps, the racerback may be the answer to your prayers. This bra is excellent if you have small or sloped shoulders that cause your straps to fall down constantly or want to diminish any strap sightings under your 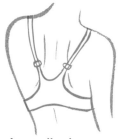 tank tops. Racerbacks have a front closure and typically plunge very low in between the breasts. Another option is the convertible bra.

MINIMIZER

Presto chango, this bra is like magic! A minimizer redistributes fullness. It tucks a bit of your breast tissue toward your underarms, resulting in the appearance of smaller breasts and less boob out front. This can help you enormously when your button-front shirts, well, never button.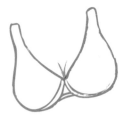

True Lingerie Story:

Mother Knows Best

My mom always "supported" my changing body size and image by buying me fancy, fun bras. Through my younger years of being overweight and staring into those tall boutique mirrors hating myself, she would be right by my side...grabbing the closest DDD she could get her hands on. When I wanted her to share in my loathing, she would keep piling more supersensual underwires onto the changing room chair. When I became a confident athlete in my thirties, she joined the show! I encouraged her to shun her old cotton panties and go for the sexy satin Felinas. To this day, she's always the central figure in my annual bra pilgrimage.

—*Heather G.*, 36F

Hot Mama

Pregnant or nursing moms need not despair—attractive nursing bras do exist! Elle Macpherson Intimates and Le Mystère both make stylish yet practical pieces that won't sacrifice your fashion sensibilities. Bella Materna also makes beautiful bras and loungewear you will want to use long after your baby is out of diapers. Look for microfiber fabric that wicks away moisture; avoid cotton bras, which become misshapen and uncomfortably damp. For sleeping, buy a pullover-style bra, sans hooks for comfort. Get properly fitted and support your girls during daytime outings. It will make you look and feel better.

SOFT

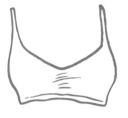

Not diggin' your underwire bra diggin' into you? The soft bra is a favorite among smaller-breasted women who don't feel they need an underwire bra, or women who simply can't tolerate one. This style comes in a huge variety of materials, from basic cotton and microfiber to frilly lace. The soft bra is becoming increasingly popular in a contour style because the light padding provides great shape under clothes, without the underwire. If you want more support, look for a snug band that hooks in the back. The one-piece, hookless, pullover styles are typically more about comfort and less about support.

SPORTS

You got game? This is your gym bag essential. This bra minimizes the movement of your breasts during rigorous exercise. You can find sports bras in different materials and styles. If you're

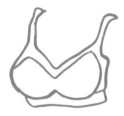

thinking "uniboob," think again. Styling has come a long way since the inception of this style. They are available with underwire for maximum support, in simple cotton styles, or with thick elastic and moisture-wicking material for lengthy workouts. Some busty gals who don't want to work out in an underwire layer their sports bras for extreme support. Spectators agree that this indispensable piece is for sports play only—not foreplay, or it's Game Over.

STICK-ON

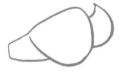

Stuck with a backless dress and no bra? Stick it on! There are several styles available on the market. You can find slim stick-on silicone breast covers with an attachment between the breasts for a bit of cleavage. There are also versions that have a contour-front bra with stick-on wings that adhere to your sides to offer a bit of support. Some feature round, oval or U-shaped tabs that adhere to the breasts and hold them up independently. Choose the style based on the shape of top or dress you plan to wear. Make no mistake: these are not supportive bras. However, they can provide a little shape and nipple control for backless outfits (preferably snug-fitting tops). If you need a backless bra but can't bear the idea of sticking it on, Maidenform has introduced one that has nothing sticky about it, except you must wear straps with it.

The Price You Pay

Like a pair of jeans that sells for twenty dollars and a pair that sells for two hundred dollars, bra pricing runs the gamut between cheap and luxurious. So what are the differences between a twenty-dollar bra and one that costs one hundred dollars? Usually, fit and construction. A more expensive bra has typically passed more hurdles than an Olympic runner when it comes to fittings. Manufacturers focus on the engineering and technology of the fabric and fit to ensure shapely and well-supported consumers. Pricey bras generally offer higher quality and better constructed detailing, such as hand-cut lace and embellishments. Upgraded fabrics—such as soft and comfy Italian microfiber, known for its special moisture-wicking properties—are used in some pricier pieces. Ultimately, if the bra fits, is comfortable and looks fantastic on you, it's worth it. No matter what the price tag says.

Panties

BRIEF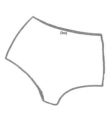

Also known as Granny Panties, these underpants do have their place. This modest style offers full coverage front and back, and some are downright pretty nowadays, in pleasing patterns and prints or embellished with lace and bows. However, briefs typically have a higher rise in the front, some up to the belly button, and back (read: don't wear these with your low-rise jeans or on date nights). Wear these under dresses with ease.

BOYSHORT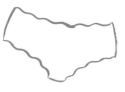

These cheeky little panties show that you can have a little more coverage and still be sexy. They come in a variety of shapes and styles, mostly low rise on the hip. From the front they look like shorts, with ample coverage. Yet in the back they may reveal a lot of booty, a little bit of booty or no booty at all, depending on the style. They are also deliciously comfortable and avert the panty-line problem. A variation is a thong-style short; it looks like a short in front, with a thick, thong-style back. Sassy!

On the Rise

When we speak about "rise," we are referring to how high a panty comes up on your hips and tummy. Low rise, for example, should just cover your cheek cleavage. Mid-rise panties should hit about halfway between your belly button and your bikini line. High-rise panties can hit anywhere between mid rise and your navel. You can find thongs, bikinis, boyshorts or pretty much any type of panty in any rise.

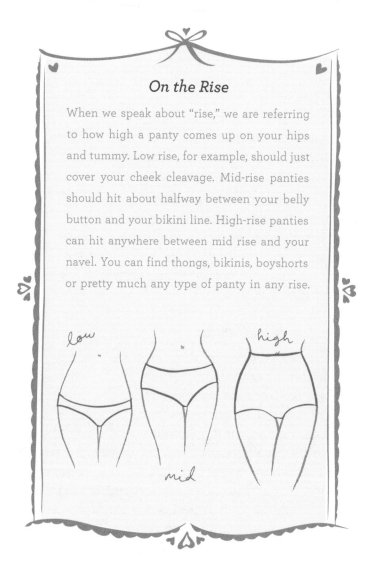

low

high

mid

BIKINI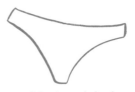

With the wild popularity of the bikini swimsuit in the 1960s, this panty has been de rigueur for decades. Traditionally, it provides moderate coverage in the front and back, with high-cut legs. Bikinis can fit perfectly under low-rise pants or offer coverage up to the belly button, depending on the cut and style. String bikinis are a variation that has skimpier coverage in the front and back, with ribbon-size sides. Tip: look for bikinis with a seam up the center of your derriere to give a rounder bottom shape under clothes.

BRAZILIAN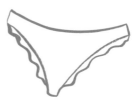

This term means more than a thorough waxing. It's a panty style particularly loved by those who want to elongate their legs or visually slim their thighs. (Think dance skirt sashaying as you samba across the room.) These panties are cut high on the thigh and are available in both bikini and thong. Great if you want a little more coverage everywhere without sacrificing sexiness.

TANGA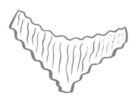

These exotically named panties are a nice compromise between a thong and a bikini. A tanga has roughly an equal amount of material in the back as in the front, leaving you more exposed in back with nice coverage in front. This style avoids panty lines and gives a little more coverage to those who don't do thongs.

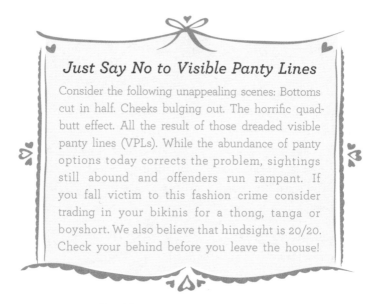

Just Say No to Visible Panty Lines

Consider the following unappealing scenes: Bottoms cut in half. Cheeks bulging out. The horrific quad-butt effect. All the result of those dreaded visible panty lines (VPLs). While the abundance of panty options today corrects the problem, sightings still abound and offenders run rampant. If you fall victim to this fashion crime consider trading in your bikinis for a thong, tanga or boyshort. We also believe that hindsight is 20/20. Check your behind before you leave the house!

THONG

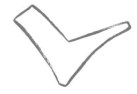

Love 'em or hate 'em, these little scraps of material do their job by eradicating VPLs. The thong typically is made with a small triangle of material in the front and just a thin piece —little more than a string—that rests between your cheeks. The absence of fanny coverage ensures the absence of panty lines.

G-STRING

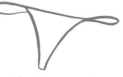

This is the tiniest thong you can imagine. And we didn't think of it first: it originated among the tribal people from thousands of years ago. A small triangle of material is in front, with strings running up your cheek cleavage and across your hips.

Hosiery and Stockings

PANTYHOSE

This mid-century invention "liberated" women from the garter belt. The hosiery covers you from waist to toes. The panty portion varies: it can be reinforced and darker shaded, give the illusion of lacy panties or be completely sheer. If you're going to wear sandals, choose the seamless, sheer-toed variety or the styles made specifically for peep-toe shoes, which leave your toes free.

CONTROL HOSIERY

We believe in self-control when necessary. Control-top pantyhose sucks in your tummy and holds up your hose. This style is usually preferred, as it discourages the "saggy-crotch syndrome," which makes you pull and tug at your bottom all day long. Some control-top hosiery sucks in your thighs and hips. Another style, made popular by SPANX, is pantyhose sans feet, which gives you an allover smooth look under pants or a long skirt.

TIGHTS

Great for fall and cooler days, tights are also a fabulous way to make a fashion statement or add color to an outfit. The opaque hosiery is made with a higher denier, or thickness, in fabrics such as nylon, cotton and wool.

FISHNETS

Ladies, make no mistake—men love these. Depending on the rest of your outfit, fishnets lend a look of sophistication (if paired with a demure or classic dress) or seduction (if worn with a supershort skirt and stilettos). These sexy stockings are meshed material in a diamond-shaped pattern, which can be tightly or loosely woven so less or more skin is exposed.

THIGH HIGHS

Thigh highs usually come in two varieties: those that require garter belts and those that "stand alone." The former type has a soft top, typically of lace or nylon, that stays up with the help of a garter belt. The latter has a bit of silicone around the top band that grabs on to your thigh and won't fall down on the job. Either way, a peek at the top of these is a surefire turn-on.

GARTER

This petite piece of lingerie is best known as something a groom retrieves from his bride's thigh and throws to his pals in the wedding hall. But the iconic symbol of marriage also serves a purpose: they can keep stockings up as well. Garters are usually embellished, lacy little things.

GARGER BELT ✿ 💎 👠

What began as a workhorse to hold up hose has become a garment often used for fun and foreplay. A garter belt is a "belt" that fastens around your waist or hips. It traditionally has four (or more, or fewer) straps with hooks and clips that attach to your thigh highs. You can find simple, flat-front garter belts for daily wear, frilly lace ones that match your favorite bra and

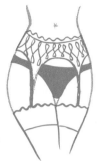

panty set or waist cincher–style belts that provide equal amounts coquetry and tummy control. Garter belt virgins should try before they buy; some can be very difficult to fasten.

HOW TO ATTACH A GARTER BELT TO STOCKINGS

Putting on a garter belt and stockings can be a simple exercise or a twenty-minute workout involving sweating and cursing. This is definitely a case of practice making perfect. Follow this guide step-by-step and, with a little care and patience, you'll soon master the garter belt.

1. Purchase a good model. Garter belts are easiest to attach when they have a metal "receiver" with an indentation and an adjoining rubber or plastic bit to insert into it. The stockings are placed between these two gizmos, which hold them in place. Thriftier models, made exclusively from plastic, can be infinitely more difficult to attach as the plastic bends easily. We suggest purchasing a well-made quality model. Believe us, it will be worth it.

2 Choose your stockings. Stockings for garter belts are the traditional type—they don't stay up on their own. Thigh highs with silicone on the top (aka "stay ups") stay up on their own accord, as they have a silicone band around the top. However, the silicone makes the band thicker and can interfere with garter belt fastening. We suggest novices use stockings specifically for garter belts. Fishnets are another option. Seamed hosiery is exceptionally sexy; just make sure the seams are centered and run straight up the backs of your legs.

3 Put on your stockings. Start by gathering them, as you would socks, down to the toe. Then gently slide them over your toes, feet and legs.

4 Put on your garter belt. Most of them fasten in the back with one or several hooks, although some slide on or zip up, depending on the style. You will have two straps in front, one hanging in front of each thigh, and two straps in back. The garter belt should sit somewhere between your natural waist and your hips, depending on your preference and the width of the belt. We recommend wearing it right under your belly button—it covers up any tummy pooch and seems to be the most flattering place in general. If you don't have much of a waist, wear it at waist height to create the appearance of one.

5 Attach the garter belt fasteners to your stockings. Start with the strap on one side in the back. Remove the rubber clasp from the metal or plastic fastener (slide it up the channel so the rubber bit comes loose). Slide the top of the stocking under the fastener and replace the rubber clasp, pushing the stocking into place and sliding the rubber bit back down the channel to lock it in place. Give the stocking a little tug to make sure it is attached. Next, attach the other back strap. The straps should be somewhat centered on your thighs. If you need to shift your stockings a bit to gain symmetry, now is the time to do it!

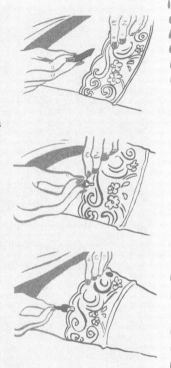

6 Attach the front fasteners, centering them on each thigh.

7 Panties are optional, but if you choose to wear them, put them on now. You can then easily remove them without removing the garter belt. This provides easy bathroom access during dinner—and easy access for your man after dinner.

8 Voilà! You are finished. Now go strut your stuff in your steamy getup.

Other Key Underthings

CAMISOLE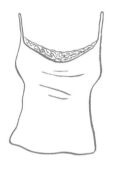

This is one of the most versatile pieces of lingerie to reveal itself in years—literally. The camisole now peeks out from under everything, including skimpy summer tops, plunging necklines and business suits. It is basically a tank top that you layer, like a slip, under your clothing. These pieces provide warmth, discretion and style; they also create smooth lines. Adjustable straps are handy for daily wear and built-in shelf bras are great for support if you wear them without a bra. The wide range of fabric, colors and styles makes them collectible. You can never have too many of them. Before you shop, have an idea of what you want and need: neutrals or colors, smooth or lacy, loose or body-hugging, style of neckline.

SLIP (AKA FULL SLIP)

A full slip will keep that dress from clinging to your derriere or letting the sun shine through thin material. Slips are layering undergarments of varying lengths intended to be worn under a dress. But they can also be layered as edgy fashion statements. This piece is usually made of nylon or a "slippery" material and comes with thin shoulder straps.

HALF SLIP

The half sister of the full slip is worn under skirts and is available in varying lengths.

Lounging and More

DRESSING GOWN/ROBE ⚙ ⌒ ✿ ◈ ⟋

The terms *dressing gown* and *robe* are interchangeable. However, *robe* tends to conjure up something soft, fluffy and warm, and *dressing gown* evokes images of Hollywood starlets in long and slinky numbers from bygone days. The point is, you use it to cover up after your shower or when you answer the door for the cable guy. Robes come in most imaginable fabrics, from bamboo modal to lightweight silk and cottons, and are available in varying lengths.

BABYDOLL ✿ ◈ ⟋

This innocently named piece of lingerie can be sweet or sensuous, for sleep or sex. The A-line-shaped top barely covers your bottom and often comes with a matching panty. Some styles have a split up the middle, exposing your midsection.

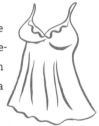

CHEMISE ⚙ ⌒ ✿ ◈ ⟋

A chemise may be the most flattering item in your lingerie drawer. This variable-length nightie is usually made of slinky and forgiving fabric that drapes simply and beautifully over a multitude of "problem areas," including ample tummies, thighs and derrieres. Have fun with this one—choose from solids or prints, simple or lacy, classic or chic styles. Made for sleep or play.

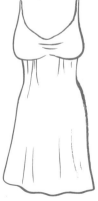

NIGHTGOWN

While some of us sleep in the buff, many enjoy slipping into a little something at nighttime, like a nightgown. They are typically long, fluid, calf- or ankle-length gowns made from silk, satin, lace, cotton or anything luxurious. A peignoir set is a nightgown paired with a long dressing gown. Brides and divas alike enjoy the allure of these pieces.

TEDDY

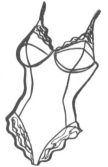

If the term *teddy* conjures up cat-eye eyeliner or leg warmers, don't be alarmed. It's a piece of lingerie that fades in and out of fashion. But one thing is for sure: men never tire of unsnapping it. This one-piece garment fastens at the crotch. It may be loose fitting, with tap-style shorts and a blousy camisole top, or it may be tight, made from stretchy fabric with a thong bottom and a bra-style top—or any variation in between. You'll also find shapewear teddies, which are both practical and attractive. Hello low-rise jeans, goodbye belly!

TAP PANTS

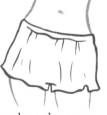

They're flippy and flirty and yes, you can tap in them; they were actually developed for dancing. But, these adorable bottoms have additional functions. Frequently worn in place of a slip under short skirts or dresses, tap pants also double as sleep and loungewear. The loose-fitting short shorts are made of silk or satiny material and usually have slits on the sides. You can wear them with or without underwear. Ooh la la!

Special Items

CORSET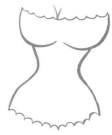

Not just a suction device, but also a saucy accessory! Molder of bodies and shaper of waists, this nineteenth-century invention is typically a heavily boned piece with laces or hooks running up the front and/or back. A corset may or may not have underwire cups and usually reaches from just over the bust to over the hips. Generally, this item pushes your goods up. It can be more "industrial" for those who truly want that wasp-waisted or hourglass shape. It can also be gorgeously lacy and detailed, appropriate to wear for bedroom fun or teamed with jeans or a skirt as an outerwear piece. A corset sometimes has garter attachments. Wear with coordinating panties and strike a pose.

WAIST CINCHER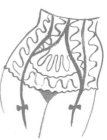

Need a little nip and tuck around the waist? Corset-style waist cinchers fit under the bust and often come with garter belt attachments. These are great for camouflaging a little tummy while adding drama to your boudoir outfit. They're also a good choice if you can't find a corset large enough to accommodate your breasts: you can just wear your bra and add the cincher for effect. You typically combine these with a bra and panty set.

BUSTIER 🌸 💎 👠

First, let's get this straight: *bustier* is pronounced "boo-stee-ay." It's basically a bra with metal or plastic boning that extends down the rib cage, often to the waist or hips. These breast-enhancing shapers are functional, or fun for when you're feeling frisky. There are several variations. A long-line version, which

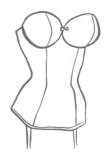

extends to, or over, the hips, is ideal underneath a clingy dress or for the bride who needs some extra support and shaping. A merry widow is a bustier with a built-in garter belt. Bustiers come with or without straps.

SHAPEWEAR 🪝 🌸 💎 👠

Shapewear is truly a girl's best friend! This category comprises all items intended to be worn underneath your clothing to control or tame trouble areas. Typically made from a blend of nylon, elastane (better known as Lycra or spandex) or cotton, there are myriad options when it comes to shapewear, depending on the designer and the amount of control you need. You can find light-, medium- or firm-control garments with different levels of compression to smooth bulges and give problem areas a more taut appearance. Here are a few places where we tend to need a little help.

Upper Body/Midsection

- High-waist brief: Extends over your tummy up to your bra band. Provides suction and shaping for your tummy and bottom.

- Camisole with built-in suction: Flattens your abdomen and tummy. Available with or without built-in bra.

- Waist cincher: Squeezes your midsection and creates a more defined waist.

Lower Body

- Control-top pantyhose: Control your tummy, booty and, sometimes, thigh area.

- Shorts: Tighten your thighs and derriere, and create smooth lines.

- Footless tights: Offer extra suction in the thigh and tummy.

The Whole Enchilada

- High-waist control-top pantyhose: These reach up to the bra line for total body tightening.

- Bodysuit: Think one-piece swimsuit. It has built-in bra and panty, keeping everything smooth and firm.

- High-waist thigh-slimming shorts: The waist extends up to your bra.

We like shapewear from Body Nancy Ganz, Body Wrap, SPANX, Wacoal, Va Bien and Berkshire Hosiery.

Women of America,
you need to rise up and
get a proper bra fitting!

- OPRAH WINFREY

CHAPTER 4

Sizing Matters

A PERFECT FIT FOR EVERY BODY TYPE

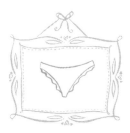

Fit is number one on your list when it comes to buying lingerie you love. If you're bulging out in the wrong spots or you're not making the most of your God-given assets, then you need to reassess what's right for you. After all, lingerie is all about feeling good and looking sexy. The basics of great-fitting lingerie are simple:

- Choosing pieces that complement your body type and height
- Selecting lingerie that complements your breast shape and size
- Establishing your bra size, ideally with professional help
- Considering panty style
- Picking panties that complement your derriere

True Lingerie Story:

From Smashed to Smashing

One weekend a twenty-four-year-old woman came into my shop, Bellefleur Lingerie. She was trying on pajamas and expressed how she loathed shopping for lingerie because of her awkward size. She said she was a 34A and could never find bras that fit her properly. I convinced her to do a bra fitting as she was clearly in the wrong size. Much to her surprise, she was a full 34C cup; she had been squeezing her beautiful breasts into tiny cups that smashed and distorted them. She tried on a sexy 34C lace demi-cup bra, let out a gasp and glowed at the reflection in the mirror. After spending four hundred dollars, she left the shop feeling beautiful and excited about her body shape and the fit of her new lingerie.

—*Jennifer C.*, 34B

Body Type

Women come in all shapes and sizes. It's what makes us unique, special and eternally frustrated when we can't fit into the latest designer trend. Lingerie is the same way—you can try to put your body into the same thing that everyone else is wearing, but the end result is not always the same. For example, if you are a 34A your push-up bra will surely make you look perky and perhaps a little more busty. Whereas a 34DD in the same style bra may look a little more porn-star. (Not to say that a little porn-star is a bad thing.) The point is, the same style bra can look completely different on two different women.

You may already know your shape, your assets and your figure challenges. If not, here is a list of some general body types and challenges. Your body might have characteristics in more than one category.

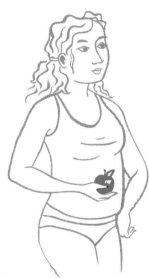

APPLE

Your top half is proportionately bigger than your bottom half. You typically have a larger bust and tummy, a smaller booty, and slim hips and legs. You gain your weight at and above the waist. The best-fitting lingerie for you, Apple, tends to accentuate your ample bosom and slim legs while discreetly covering your tummy.

Sans clothes: Wear babydolls. They'll show off your nice legs and small booty. These fluttery, A-line-shaped chemises barely cover your behind. Avoid any that split up the middle and show your tummy. Another option is a corset. It plays up your assets by boosting boobs. Thigh highs look fantastic on your slim legs. Pair them with the corset for a night of naughtiness.

Under clothes: Invest in a good bra that lifts and separates, creating a waist and a longer torso. Consider a waist cincher or piece of shapewear that smoothes your torso and belly bulges. A one-piece bodysuit with a built-in bra and snap panty offers lots of control and visually eliminates unsightly rolls.

Don't: Wear tight-fitting camisoles or chemises that accentuate your midsection.

PEAR

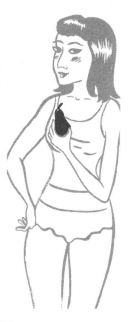

Your bottom half is proportionately bigger than your top half. You may have small, teardrop-shaped breasts, a flat stomach, and a full bottom and hips. Your hips are often wider than your shoulders, and your thighs are curvy. Skinny jeans may be your worst enemy. Pears can create proportion by drawing attention upward with specialty bras or camisoles that are push-up or patterned, colored or sheer.

Sans clothes: Wear an A-line chemise or gown that hits below the booty to create sleek lines. Pair a sheer camisole or bra with a boyshort. It will highlight your upper assets while providing coverage for your curvaceous caboose.

Under clothes: A little padding in your bra can go a long way. Adding some volume and shape to your upper body will create more balance and proportion with your bottom. Invest in some control capris or shorts to smooth any bottom bulges under tight-fitting pants, dresses or skirts. Some shapewear can take nearly a whole size off your bottom!

Don't: Wear ruffles around hips and booty. This will only make those areas appear larger.

HOURGLASS

You are a lucky lady. You have the much-sought-after shape: a proportionate top and bottom with a smaller waist. You gain weight evenly and have fewer problems than women with other body types do when trying to find clothing that fits well.

Sans clothes: Show off your curves by wearing bra and panty sets and body-hugging teddies or chemises.

Under clothes: Pay close attention to any pulling or gapping in your clothing. Layer a camisole beneath your button-front shirt and leave it unbuttoned at the top, where it doesn't close properly. Or wear control panties with your snug trousers to eliminate any muffin-top effect (hip or abdomen spillage).

Don't: Wear oversize or baggy tops that lack structure and hide your lovely figure. You may look heavier when you don't show off your waist.

SPORTY

You are typically referred to as having a "sporty" physique. You may be small- or large- boned, but you have a solid torso with little waist definition. Your goal is to create visual curves with your lingerie.

Sans clothes: Wear a two-piece set, such as a cropped camisole with a thong, in dark or contrasting colors, to give you the illusion of curves.

Under clothes: Wear a foundation bra that fits well, to separate your breasts and create some curves. Think push up and out!

Don't: Wear a tight-fitting nightgown. It will make you look like a sausage—and not in an appetizing way.

Height

TALL GALS

It's difficult to find the right fit for your body. Most clothing is cut too small for you, many tops are too short and nightgowns look like camisoles.

Sans clothes: Wear gowns or chemises that are long. They look incredible on you—work that height! You also look hot in bra and panty sets and garter belts.

Under clothes: If you are wearing tight-fitting clothing, make sure any bulges or trouble areas are firmly controlled by your undergarments. Pay close attention to your hips and tummy, and invest in a high-top panty that sucks in that whole area. Bigger is *not* better in these places.

Don't: Wear babydolls (unless they split down the front) or extra-short chemises. They will look like blouses on you and will distort your proportions.

PETITE GALS

Being petite makes finding the right scale of clothing a challenge. Lucky for you, most lingerie is cut on the small side. And with lingerie, less can certainly be more!

Sans clothes: Wear camisole and panty sets, and bra and panty sets. You look adorable in all things skimpy. A tie-side thong and sheer bra expose more skin, playing up your body.

Under clothes: Be sure to accentuate your positive attributes, be it a curvy booty or perky bust. Wear well-fitting undergarments to look your best in clothing.

Don't: Wear long nightgowns that cover you completely or anything baggy and shapeless. This will make you look frumpy and shrink your size further, instead of accentuating the hot little body you have.

Breast Size and Shape

AMPLE

Your breasts are a constant force, concern or consideration in your life. You often feel there are no bras you love in your size and that you couldn't possibly wear what those 34B ladies are wearing. Support is key for you full-busted gals. If you're a full C cup or larger, you should be wearing something that hugs your bust and offers some support. Embrace those curves and show them off. Remember, people pay good money for an ample bosom. Appreciate your girls!

Sans clothes: Find a chemise or bra that is supportive and cleavage revealing. Wear a bra under a nightie. You'll feel more supported and also more confident about the ensemble.

Under clothes: Get a bra fitting (never mind about modesty!) and wear a supportive bra in your size. Stop wearing a bra that's two sizes too small because you want to be a C cup. The best thing you can do for your body is to wear the right size!

Don't: Wear loose-fitting nightgowns or triangle-shaped bra tops with no stretch. They lend no support—physically or emotionally.

SMALL

You may feel that your small bust does not warrant a bra. Perhaps you don't feel you can wear all the fun lingerie that the ladies with bigger breasts can exhibit. Sometimes less is more! Enjoy the fact that you don't have to look for support in every top you wear.

Sans clothes: Rejoice that you look ravishing in barely there lingerie. With support being a nonissue, small-breasted girls look hot in sheer and lacy demi-style bras, camisoles and chemises. Show off what you've got. Ruffles and ruching are also your friends and will help add volume if you want to look like you have even more to offer.

Under clothes: Buy a push-up bra or something with a little padding to make your shirt or blouse fit better. Invest in some silicone inserts that fit into any bra for some added va va voom.

Don't: Wear that push-up bra for hanky-panky. It may look great under clothes, but when the clothes come off, padding is a bust! Avoid premolded tops that are baggy or look too big.

UNEVEN

While nearly all women have a discrepancy in breast size, some women have a half cup or more difference. This makes bra shopping somewhat tedious at best and, at worst, an unpleasant experience. Here is a rule to live by: *the bigger breast wins!*

Sans clothes: Wear stretch lace bras and tops that do not accentuate the difference, but do accommodate both breast sizes.

Under clothes: Wear bras that fit the larger breast best. It's better to have some room on one side than to be squished on the other. Contour-cup bras are the best choice for you: they create a visual symmetry under clothes and allow harmonious coexistence between you and your breasts. If there is a large discrepancy, add a silicone insert so the girls will be on equal ground.

Don't: Buy soft-cup or cotton bras, which only accentuate the problem.

Petite Busts

Small bust? Don't despair! These tips come from petite-lingerie and -bra specialist extraordinaire Ellen Shing, of Lula Lu in San Mateo, California (see "Shop Talk" appendix for contact info).

1. Many small-busted women become accustomed to not filling their bra cups, resulting in either gaps at the top of the cups or empty space inside the cups. If you are wearing an A cup and encounter these issues, look for AA-cup styles that will fit your body type better. Your bra cup should be touching your skin, not standing away from your body.

2. AA- and A-cup women don't necessarily need to wear underwire bras. In some cases, especially when you are wearing a fitted top, the underwires on a small bust can appear as "smiley faces" under the breasts. An assortment of soft-cup bras that look great and are extremely comfortable are available in small sizes.

3. Enjoy your small bust and try bras with various levels of padding. Who cares if anyone's wondering if you had a boob job! Sometimes a little false advertising under a sweater or dress can make you feel much more confident. Other times, you may prefer to wear a bra that reflects your true size—because *it* looks fantastic, too.

PLUS-SIZE

If you wear more than a 38-inch band, it may be challenging to find anything that has any style or color. Don't despair! More and more bra manufacturers are getting the picture: full-figured ladies want beautiful bras, too. Thanks to companies and brands such as Prima Donna and Chantelle, and retail shops such as Lane Bryant, the voluptuous can now celebrate their busts with beautifully intricate and supportive bras.

Sans clothes: Wear beautiful, lacy underwire bras that reflect your personality. If you love colors, go for it. Make sure the band fits properly and is supportive.

Under clothes: Wear smooth, contour-cup bras that lift and separate the girls. This will give you a curvy figure and balance any bottom-heavy proportions.

Don't: Be afraid to show off your décolletage with confidence. You've got 'em, so flaunt 'em.

Bra Fit

It's cliché but true: one thing you can count on in life is that things will change. This applies not only to your relationships and waistline, but also to your bra size. In fact, your bra size may change several times throughout your lifetime because of various factors, such as weight gain or loss, surgical procedures, hormonal changes related to health, birth control pills, pregnancy, menopause and age.

When trying to determine your true bra size, you need to throw all preconceived notions about your body, breast size and bra styles out the window. You may think you're flat or oddly shaped. Or you may feel that bras are always too small, too big, uncomfortable or not cut right for your body. You may think you have back fat, or underarm fat, and that your clothes don't fit correctly and it looks like a bulgy mess. The fact is that you're just wearing the wrong size bra.

Discovering your correct bra size can be a liberating experience, both physically and emotionally. A supportive bra that fits well can create visual symmetry for pear shapes, define a waist for apple shapes, add curves to sporty shapes and give overall aid in how your clothes fit and drape. Physically, you will be wearing something that is comfortable, looks fabulous and requires no tugging or pulling. Emotionally, you will be relieved because you know you are supported, look good and feel great. You'll be more confident no matter what you're wearing— and that's always sexy.

Finding the right size bra isn't magic or rocket science. It's about getting baseline measurements and choosing the right styles. The best way to find your proper size is to make a trip to your local lingerie shop or to a department store, such as Nordstrom, that employs fit specialists. Being fit for a bra is a quick and painless venture, even for shy ladies or bra novices. An expert bra-fitting specialist will be able to measure you, assess your correct size and suggest different styles that fit your particular shape.

Bra fitting can be a very intimate experience. You are taking your top off and letting your guard down. Don't be modest. Remember that fitters are professionals who want you to look and feel better. And yours aren't the first set of breasts they've seen.

True Lingerie Story:

The Day I Met Juliette

I've had back problems since I was thirteen, when I first developed a chest. When I was eighteen and my breasts were quite substantial, the pain worsened. I did everything I could think of to strengthen my back for twenty years, including chiropractic, swimming, yoga and Pilates—nothing helped. I resorted to painkillers to try to alleviate the discomfort.

Finally, at thirty-three, when I was living in London, I had a proper bra fitting. I'd read about Rigby & Peller, the official brassiere makers for the queen. I figured if the shop was good enough for the queen, it was good enough for me. The women in Rigby & Peller were serious about their bra fittings. They had me in a dressing room and my top off within thirty seconds. They took one look at my bra and said, "No wonder you've had back pain." Before I could say Mary Poppins, they'd popped me into a new bra.

The whole thing took about two minutes. I stood there staring in the mirror. I was used to these Sherman-tank styles, wearing a size 36DD. This bra was a red, lacy number and it was a 32F. The name of the bra was Juliette. I loved her. I bought as many bras as I could afford. I've never had back pain since.

—*Maile R.*, **32F**

DO IT YOURSELF:
HOW TO DETERMINE YOUR BRA SIZE

If you are unable to get a personal fitting, you can determine your bra size yourself. Keep in mind that not all measurements are set in stone, especially when it comes to cup size. (Manufacturers do not standardize.) Due to the variety of breast shapes, sometimes measurement is not the only indicator of size. However, here are some specific guidelines to help you determine your bra size with some basic measurements.

You will need a soft tape measure and an unpadded underwire bra.

Put on the bra and make sure the band is horizontal and firm across your back, not riding up between your shoulder blades.

STEP 1. BAND MEASUREMENT & SIZE

Measure around the band of your bra while holding the tape snugly under your bust. Add 4 or 5 to this number, whichever results in an even number.

Examples: If you measure 29 around, that translates into a 33–34 band; so you wear a 34. If you measure 32, that becomes 36–37; so you need a 36" band. For 1/2 measurements, round down; for 3/4 measurements, round up. For instance, if you measure 29½, that becomes 29. If you measure 29¾, that becomes 30.

Measurement _____ + 4" or 5" = _____

Enter your band size here: _____

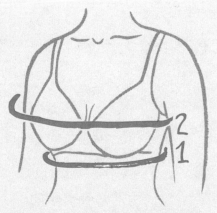

STEP 2. BREAST MEASUREMENT

Measure around the fullest part of your bust, horizontally across your back. Leave the tape a little looser this time; do not squeeze it tight. This measurement will be used to determine your cup size.

Enter your breast measurement here: _____

STEP 3. DO THE MATH

Subtract your band size from your breast measurement.

Enter the difference here: _____

STEP 4. CUP SIZE

Using the following chart, determine your cup size.

Enter your cup size here: _____

CUP SIZE CHART

If difference between band size and breast measurement is:

Less than 1	AA cup
1	A cup
2	B cup
3	C cup
4	D cup
5	DD cup or E cup
6	DDD cup or F cup
7	DDDD cup or G cup

STEP 5. BRA SIZE

Enter your band size, then your cup size: _____

Voilà! This is your correct bra size.

Quick Size Fix: The most common bra faux pas is wearing a band size that's too big and a cup size that's too small. If you are wearing a 36B and it seems okay but not perfect, try a 34C (go down a band size and up a cup size). The cup size relates directly to the band size, so, yes, you really *could* be a C cup. C cups come in all sizes, as do A, B, D and Es.

Your breasts should sit somewhere between your shoulders and your elbows. The higher the better! Keep that in mind when trying on bras. If your breasts are low riding, the bra is probably not supportive enough.

A properly fitted bra will do the following:

- Be supportive
- Not rub or leave red marks
- Sit horizontally around your back
- Have a good-fitting underwire that nearly comes to your armpits, without cutting into your breast tissue or creating bulges
- Possess a middle saddle (the connecting material between your breasts) that sits flat against your sternum
- Comfortably fasten on the first (loosest) set of hooks and eyes when new. This gives your bra lasting power: you can tighten it by advancing to the second or third set when it stretches out.

New Girls on the Block

Those of you who purchased your bountiful breasts may be confused about the fit of your bras. The doctor may have told you that you are one size, yet you may fit into an entirely different size. The rub is that your breasts look round and supported in nearly everything you put on, so how can you tell what fits? Go to your local lingerie boutique and be professionally fitted. Staff can tell you where the underwire should be hitting your body.

GETTING IT ON: HOW TO PUT ON YOUR BRA

An ill-adjusted bra can feel just as uncomfortable as the wrong size bra. Once you have determined your accurate size and are shopping for the perfect bra, be sure to put it on correctly. Start by putting your arms through the shoulder straps and securing the bra in the back, on the loosest or middle hook. If you are unable to hook the bra in the back, you may fasten it in the front and slide the band around until the hooks are centered on your back; then put your arms through the shoulder straps. Adjust the straps so the band fits snugly and horizontally around your rib cage; it shouldn't ride up your back or in between your shoulder blades. Next, pull any side breast tissue (under your arms) into the cup, making sure the underwire is resting firmly on your rib cage (on both sides). If you have very full breasts and have a small amount of spillage in the cleavage area, take your fingers and gently adjust the fabric to achieve a smooth line. You can do this by running a finger up each side where the material meets your breast. Congratulations, now you have a comfortably fitting bra!

WEAR AND TEAR

The average life span of a bra you wear daily is roughly six months. If you have large breasts and the bra has to do some heavy lifting, you may cycle through them faster. If you rarely purchase lingerie and can't remember the last time you bought a new bra, we recommend buying four new bras at a time. Four bras should give you at least two years of daily wear before you have to replenish.

Postsurgery Bras

Whether you have had a lumpectomy or a mastectomy, finding a bra that fits correctly may feel like a challenge. With a lumpectomy you may notice that one breast is a slight to full cup size different than the other. The bigger breast wins. Choose a contour bra that has fiberfill, to camouflage the smaller breast while supporting both breasts and creating a symmetrical shape under clothing.

If you have had a partial or full mastectomy, you may choose a prosthetic insert (typically silicone) to be worn inside your bra cup. Department stores, such as Nordstrom, offer fitting services in their lingerie departments. If you are uncertain where to go, call your doctor's office for recommendations.

Bring your best-fitting presurgery bra to your fit appointment; this will allow the specialist to find the proper size for your body. Your bra should be snug fitting to support the weight of the insert. If you don't own a bra that fits well, don't worry; the fit specialist will take care of you.

ILL-FITTING BRAS: PROBLEMS AND SOLUTIONS

PROBLEM:	WHAT'S HAPPENING:	SOLUTIONS:
Straps fall off shoulders.	The band is too big and is sliding up your back, causing your already tightened straps to fall off. Band should sit horizontally around back, not ride up between shoulder blades.	Go down one band size and up one cup size.
Bra rides up back.	The band is too big and is sliding up your back. Band should sit horizontally around back, not ride up between shoulder blades.	Go down one band size and up one cup size.
Excess fat under arms.	Breast tissue runs nearly under your arms and a too-small cup will create bulges there.	Go up one or two cup sizes.

PROBLEM:	WHAT'S HAPPENING:	SOLUTIONS:
One breast is bigger than the other.	Your bra fits the smaller breast; the other breast pours out of its cup.	It is better to have room in one cup than to be overflowing from the other cup. Wear a contour cup that fits the larger breast. Go up one cup size.
Bra cup fabric wrinkles or is empty.	Your cup size may be too large if you have excess material in your bra.	Go down a cup size. Or try a different style bra, such as a demi or demi balconette, which has less cup space. If the underwire is hitting you in the proper place (nearly to your armpit), or one breast is larger than the other and is causing the problem, then you are in the correct size but wrong style bra.

ILL-FITTING BRAS: PROBLEMS AND SOLUTIONS

PROBLEM:	WHAT'S HAPPENING:	SOLUTIONS:
Band does not touch body in front. The underwire does not lie flat or touch any part of the body.	Your cup size is too small, causing the bra to sit away from your body.	Go up one cup size or maybe two. The band and underwires should sit snugly under your breasts; the middle of the bra (the saddle) should sit flat, in between your breasts. The only exception is for very petite and well-endowed women. You ladies are sometimes more difficult to fit. Consult a bra specialist at a local shop or department store.
Breasts are overflowing from cups, both above and below.	Your cup size is too small, causing a "double-boob" effect (aka quad-boob).	Go up one cup size.

PROBLEM:	WHAT'S HAPPENING:	SOLUTIONS:
Your lace bra is creating bumps under your clothes.	Wearing lace bras under clothing can create lumps and wrinkles.	Lace bras work well under button-up shirts, light or heavy sweaters and dresses. You can also find lace bras that lie so flat you can actually wear them under knits and shirts without it being too obvious. A tight, white knit shirt does require a smooth T-shirt bra, however, if you don't want any seams or lace showing.

ILL-FITTING BRAS: PROBLEMS AND SOLUTIONS

PROBLEM:	WHAT'S HAPPENING:	SOLUTIONS:
You think T-shirt bras are padded, and you don't need any extra padding.	You haven't found the right T-shirt bra!	Most T-shirt bras are contour bras, which are not padded bras. A contour bra is a bra with formed cups with the intention of being (a) perfectly shaped and smooth under clothing, (b) supportive and (c) durable. You can find T-shirt bras with padding in them, but not all T-shirt bras are padded. There is a wide variety of T-shirt bras available: some have ultrathin contouring while others are sturdier, for serious support. When shopping for a T-shirt bra, feel the lining to ensure it is not padded. Or better yet, ask for some assistance while bra shopping. You won't regret it!

PROBLEM:	WHAT'S HAPPENING:	SOLUTIONS:
Bras show through your clothing.	You need a skin-tone bra.	Nude bras are the least visible under clothing. There are, however, other attractive options out there. You can choose a pale-pink-, cream-, ivory- or chocolate-colored bra that works with your skin tone and blends under your clothing. Pick something that looks like a second skin on you and fits great.
Nipples show through your clothes when you are cold.	You need some extra fiberfill.	Wearing a contour bra is the best way to combat "nipping out" in public. Most contour bras have enough fabric to solve this problem. If you need extra protection, consider using cookies—little padded inserts that fit inside your bra cup (typically to add volume) or silicone nipple covers (see Beyond the Basics section in chapter 5).

Derriere Size and Shape

BOUNTIFUL BEHIND

Baby got back? You ample-bottomed girls can heave a sigh of relief thanks to Beyoncé, J. Lo and other full-bootied celebrities. A big booty is hip and trendy!

Sans clothes: Enjoy looking good in all styles of panties. The thong-style boyshort is a favorite, with thick sides and a thong back to show off just enough cheek while covering hips. Bikinis, Brazilian cut, thongs and G-strings all look good on you.

Under clothes: Control-top pantyhose or shorts will help create smooth lines and minimize when needed.

Don't: Wear your underwear too small or tight on the hips. It can create bulges or lumps.

SMALL OR FLAT FANNY

Others are largely unsympathetic to your complaints, but having no booty is painful because pants, jeans and trousers tend not to fit you properly. You may find you always have a little extra material in the back, which can drive you crazy. Here is your chance to retaliate—you can wear the smallest lingerie with ease!

Sans clothes: Wear itty-bitty undies to show as much of your bum as possible. Thongs are best. But if you aren't down with the thong, you can wear a snug tanga or small bikini. Ruffles and details on the back add volume and are your friends when you are being cute around the house or romping with your beau.

Under clothes: Wear a thong to create a better shape. If you like bikinis, be aware that some manufacturers make them with ruching up the back seam, which creates a little more shape.

Don't: Wear a full brief or bikini that is saggy in the bottom. Too much material + too little booty = baggy booties. That's never sexy.

Panties

There is a wide variety of panty styles on the market today (see chapter 3). No matter what your size, body type or preferences, panties should:

- Lie flat without bunching up under your clothes due to excess material

- Fit properly so they do not bind or squeeze your hips, thighs or bottom, causing bulges or red marks

- Stay in place—panties should not ride up or chafe, and should generally be comfortable

When in doubt about your panty size, try them on! You can absolutely try on underwear in a store before you buy them. For hygienic reasons, just make sure to have your own underwear on while trying on those new panties. Thongs are the best to wear, so you can actually see how the new panty will fit you.

Now you know how your lingerie should fit! Let's go on to discover the essentials every girl needs.

*If you're wearing lingerie
that makes you feel glamorous,
you're halfway there
to turning heads.*

— ELLE MACPHERSON

CHAPTER 5

Bare Essentials

HAVE YOUR BASICS COVERED

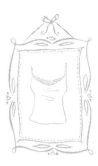

Maybe you have a drawer full of mismatched panties and bras, or one tired bra and some sad, dingy briefs. Or maybe you never have quite the right undergarment for your outer garment. Problem solved! With this simple list of essentials, you'll always have something functional and fabulous to wear underneath. If you already own a nice lingerie assortment, sort through the piles and fill the holes in your underwear drawers.

Ten Essentials
Every Girl Should Own

1. NUDE T-SHIRT BRA

This may become your go-to bra, the
one you reach for on a daily basis, as
it works well under so many types of
tops. A T-shirt bra is a contoured-cup
underwire that has enough fiberfill
to mold your breasts perfectly,

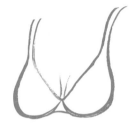

regardless of their shape or size. This bra is ideal under anything
tight and white. We suggest buying two of these indispensable
pieces, one nude and one black or in color—especially if you're the
matchy-match type and like your bra and panties to be coordinated
with your clothing. Nearly every brand offers a nude T-shirt style. We
like Chantelle, Wacoal and Le Mystère, all of which you can easily
find at any department store.

2. CONVERTIBLE/STRAPLESS BRA

How many times have you passed up
that lovely halter or spaghetti-strap
tank in your closet because you don't
have the right bra to wear underneath
it? Convertibles are a marvel of lingerie
engineering and can be worn under a
boatneck shirt, off-the-shoulder blouse,

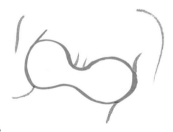

halter top or tricky-strapped summer camisole. They also work well under strapless dresses and tube tops. Bra manufacturers are becoming more creative with this style, designing them so they're both attractive and practical. Le Mystère has a wonderful push-up version that actually stays up without straps. We like the Marie Jo Avero for their pretty, flowered straps.

3. BLACK LACE BRA AND MATCHING BLACK LACE PANTY

These are the equivalent of your skinny jeans—put them on any time and feel like a million dollars. You can choose a demi, balconette or underwire bra. But it must be black lace and see-through (that means anything that shows your nipples). The same goes for the panty. It doesn't matter if you prefer bikinis or thongs, as long as they match the bra and are sheer black. Saucy! Calvin Klein and DKNY have well-made and affordable lace sets. If budget is no concern, look for Eres, Aubade or La Perla at your local boutique.

4. DATE-NIGHT BRA AND PANTY SET

This should be something out of the ordinary—special and flirty for those memorable get-lucky occasions. Try to break out of your T-shirt bra rut and buy a colorful (yes, color can be a turn-on) and lacy treat for yourself. Ask for assistance in your local lingerie shop; having someone else choose helps you expand your horizons. Tell the clerk your budget and ask her to bring you some special pieces in different styles. Get out of your comfort zone and try something new! We love Agent Provocateur for their ultraracy sets, Simone Pérèle for their beautiful color palette and Lise Charmel for their exquisite embroidered lace.

5. NUDE MICROFIBER THONG

VPLs will disappear faster than a hot fudge sundae after a three-week diet with this seamless panty. Trust us; you will want a few of these. These almost-virtual panties will not reveal

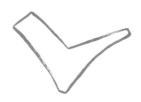

themselves through your light-colored pants, clingy trousers or skintight jeans. If you absolutely, positively can't bear to wear a thong, consider shapewear as a possible alternative (see later in this list). The best style of microfiber thong is the laser-cut, which has nearly no seams. We like the brands commando and Calvin Klein.

6. CAMISOLE

This must-have is multipurpose. Use it for layering under revealing tops, staying warm under thin blouses or keeping comfy under scratchy wool sweaters. Or, just wear it solo, as a tank top. If you're starting from scratch, find a black lace camisole you can layer under sheer tops and

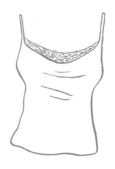

suit jackets. Another indispensable piece is a light-colored silk or modal cami. Either will keep you modest under transparent clothing, smooth out clingy shirts and keep you warm in thin blouses. We like Hanky Panky and Arianne for sophisticated, sexy lace, and Calvin Klein and Mary Green for simple, clean lines.

7. HOSIERY

Every girl should own a good pair of black tights and sheer hose. If you think nude is boring, buy a pair with a back seam to sex them up. Control top is always recommended, to avoid the "saggy crotch syndrome" we mentioned earlier. We like DKNY because they rarely run, last forever and are widely available. If you need a little suction in the rump, hip and thigh, try SPANX.

8. BIAS-CUT SILK SLIP/CHEMISE

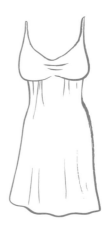

Feel glamorous lounging around your house in a comfy silk chemise rather than in his boxers or your oversize T-shirt. This multifunctional item can be worn as a slip or a nightgown. The cut is flattering on nearly every body. You can choose above-the-knee length or longer, depending on your comfort and wardrobe. We like Mary Green for the feminine silk collection, and everything Cosabella for being beautiful, trendy and well made.

9. SHAPEWEAR/CONTROL DEVICE

We all have "trouble spots," whether actual or perceived. These woven wonders will slenderize, flatten, smooth and shape where you need it most. You may try a pair of control capris to hide some cellulite under thin, white slacks. Or perhaps a pair of tummy-control panties to hold in a poochy stomach under a skimpy dress.

If excess flesh spills over your low-rise jeans, control that muffin-top effect with a pair of high-rise panties or shorts. They'll slim hips, smooth out back flab and eliminate lumps and bumps in the abdomen. We like shapewear from Body Nancy Ganz, Body Wrap, SPANX, Wacoal, Va Bien and Berkshire Hosiery.

10. ROBE

This staple provides warmth and modesty. Have it handy—who hasn't run from the bathroom to the kitchen au naturel and been caught? Invest in a warm winter robe: go for big and cozy or opt for a cotton sateen fabric or luxurious cashmere. For spring/summer and traveling, choose a short length in a lightweight fabric such as silk or cotton voile. Both tuck nicely into a weekend bag. BedHead makes beautiful cotton robes with lively prints.

Beyond the Basics

After you have your essentials covered, experiment with other items that can make your clothes fit and look better, and can make your life easier overall.

BRA WITH PRETTY STRAPS

News flash: your bra straps can be used as accessories. Show them off when you're feeling flirty or you want your skinny-strap top and bra to coexist in fashion harmony. Just remember that there's a time and place for flaunting your straps. We don't recommend letting them hang out at the office or family reunions. Our other "rule": never, never, show gray and dingy, or tattered, straps. That said, there is a huge array of pretty options and designs including lacy, textured, floral or colored straps. We like Aubade and Betsey Johnson's fancy girlie straps.

SILICONE INSERTS

Sometimes we all need a little false advertising to make that low neckline look perfect. For those of us who are cleavage challenged, a handy pair of silicone inserts can make or break an outfit. Some simply push you up, while others can add a cup size. Place them toward the bottom outer sides of your breasts, in your bra or tight top. You can find inserts filled with water, oil, air or other materials. But we like silicone best, for its natural feel (you will pass the hug test). We suggest Cleavage Cupcakes and Fashion Forms Silicone Push Up Pads.

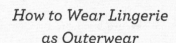

How to Wear Lingerie as Outerwear

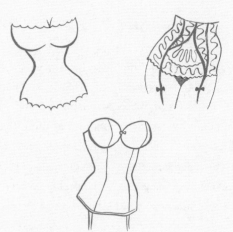

Corsets/Bustiers/Waist Cinchers: Wearing a corset or bustier in place of a fancy top or blouse is a surefire attention getter. Wear them over pencil skirts to cocktail parties, or over jeans while clubbing. Look sophisticated by pairing a simple black corset or waist cincher over a French-cuff, white button-down shirt. Very classy and drop-dead sexy.

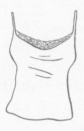

Camisoles: Camisoles are the most multipurpose piece of lingerie. Layer them under your suit jackets, your sweaters and your button-downs. Or wear them solo! Lacy, silky or comfortable cotton all look sweet teamed with jeans, skirts or slacks. Match them with your outfit or wear a contrasting color. Play with various fibers. There are even velvety fabrics for cooler weather. You can't go wrong with this style.

Full Slips: The practical, hidden slip is out—literally. Slips have been making an appearance, hanging out under dresses. Contrasting lace or satin can look classy or trashy depending on your purpose. Alternatively, if you own a beautiful ankle- or calf-length piece, why not wear it as a dress? It might just be the most flattering "dress" you own. We like a thick silk gauge and a bias cut for this trend.

NIPPLE COVERS

Always cold? Pick up some reusable nipple covers, which hide your high beams and make you feel more confident in that tight T-shirt. You can find covers that have an adhesive backing and will stick right to your nipples. Other versions include "lick and stick," which easily stay in place inside your bra. They are typically made of thin silicone or stick-on styles (think Band-Aids only better). We like DIMRS and Fashion Forms Breast Petals. For fun, try Nippies, which are one-time use stick-ons that come in different shapes and designs, including glittery stars and hearts.

True Lingerie Story:

From High to Low Beams

I never left the house in a T-shirt unless I had a sweater or layer over it. I don't need to be cold to nip out. It was constant. Padded bras didn't even work. Then I found the most ingenious product on the market: silicone nipple covers. Those covers have literally made me a new person. I now leave the house wearing whatever I want.

—*Jill A.*, 36C

HALF SLIP FOR SKIRTS

Say goodbye to static cling. You should invest in a slip that works with most of your skirt and dress lengths. Knee length is most versatile as it can be worn with anything below the knee.

CUTE PAJAMAS

Matching pj's always look more chic than frumpy, mismatched sweats. Silk, cotton, modal, solid, print—whatever. If they match and fit, you are on the right track! We like BedHead pajamas (on Oprah's "*O* List") for their funky prints and delicious cotton. And P.J. Salvage for their modal sets, which range from adorable to flirty; they're lounge-worthy and affordable.

SLIPPERS

Keep your tootsies warm and your gym socks where they belong (in your gym bag). Slippers are available from geek to chic. Express yourself with a snuggly or pretty pair, or add a little glamour to any boudoir ensemble with a pair of sassy bedroom heels. We like shopping at our local department store for the wide variety of slippers and love Jacques Levine's quintessential boudoir heels.

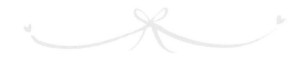

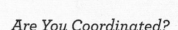

Are You Coordinated?

Bring those workhorse bras that you wear daily into your local lingerie shop and buy a bunch of coordinating bottoms. If you have black or nude bras that need panties, choose from prints, colors or lace. They don't have to match perfectly. For example, pair a black bra with a black panty trimmed in pink lace or a nude bra with a lavender panty embellished with beige bows. You can also pick up Hanky Panky's multicolor thongs, which are one size fits all and are truly comfy, with minimal or no lines. And don't miss the sale bins while getting coordinated. It's your chance to scoop up those pretty, unmatched panties at great prices.

Clean Your Drawers

Now that you know the fundamental pieces you should have on hand, you can thoroughly clean your drawers. This will aid you in assessing your lingerie deficit or surplus and in filling the holes in your lingerie chest or underwear drawers.

FIRST: Empty your underwear drawer onto your bed.

THEN: Make two piles: one of underwear that is pristine and the other of items that have snags, rips, holes, stains, funky elastic and pieces that look tired or dingy. Now toss the latter pile!

NEXT: Divide your pristine pile into lingerie you wear regularly and anything you haven't worn in the last year.

AFTER THAT: Take the pile of items you haven't worn recently and divide them into items you love and can't part with, and items that have never fit, will never fit and/or you never really liked. Now dispose of the latter pile.

FINALLY: Review this chapter. What essentials are you missing? Make a list and go shopping!

I love to wear lingerie. The problem is that men always rip it off too quickly.

- KAREN MᶜDOUGAL

CHAPTER 6

Behind Closed Doors

HOW TO DRESS FOR SEX-CESS

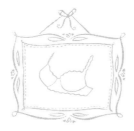

The phrase "behind closed doors" may conjure up images of clothes and/or lingerie immediately being ripped off in a frenzy of pure lust. A provocative image, yes. A scene where the excitement is prolonged and the reward sweet? Definitely not. The art of seduction does not equate with instant gratification.

Lingerie can be your secret weapon in the boudoir. Of course we hope it will incite the lust of your lover, but more than that, it will empower you. Being naked can make you feel vulnerable and, literally, exposed. You can feel comfortable while bringing out the temptress within by wearing a little lacy something that covers up your "charms." You decide what to wear (be it innocent, sassy or slutty), how much to expose and when to take it off.

The right attire can give you more confidence in your body and a sense of power in your intimate relationship. Putting on a pair of thigh highs makes him desire you even more. In short, lingerie works to your advantage.

If you're clueless or just need a few ideas to fan the flames of passion, we have some suggestions for you.

True Lingerie Story:

Is That New?

I own a few pieces of lingerie. A black bra and panty set. A red bra and panty set. A black garter belt and a red one. A few pairs of thigh highs. I switch around the pieces I am wearing based on what is clean and what coordinates. Black bra, red panty, red garter belt. Red bra, red panty, black garter belt and thigh highs. I swear my husband thinks I am wearing a new outfit every time. "Is that new?" he says. Or "That's my favorite!" he decides. Pretty tricky, huh?

—*Justine L.*, 34B

It's All about You

First, establish what type of lingerie makes you feel fabulous and turns you on. We cannot overemphasize that what makes you feel hot and sexy will no doubt make you look hot and sexy, too. If you love your stomach, show it off! If the thought of showing your thighs is repellent, wear a sleek chemise. If you haven't already, now is a good time to refer to chapter two to determine what style or styles suit you. Then review chapter four for suggestions on how to dress for your shape and body type.

And...It's All about Him

Determine what tickles your guy's fancy, and his fantasy. It may be quite different from what you have in mind. We have our own thoughts on what is sexy, as do our men. While we don't want to stereotype your guy, here are some tidy categories and guidelines to establish what, ahem, gets a rise out of him. The trick is to recognize his desires and integrate them with your needs.

A Word on Thigh Highs

Don't obsess about whether or not thigh highs make your thighs look fat. Men don't care if they pinch your thighs. They find them erotic. Period.

What Kind of Lingerie Guy Is He?

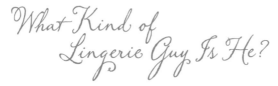

NAKED GUY

Are you stripped down immediately, with no comment on your lingerie? Your man is a minimalist. If you don't mind going buff, then do it! If you need a little somethin' somethin' to hold the girls in place, or if you feel less than scrumptious with things tottering about, wear absolutely sheer items. Choose lingerie in nude tones, with zero lace and zero frills. A sheer or near-skin-tone bra and panty set will do the trick, too. If you love lace there are lots of lovely tattoo lace options—think see-through sheer fabric with barely there embroidery.

PLAIN JANE GUY

Does your man pounce on you when he sees your daily-driver bra and bikinis? This is a no-frills man who appreciates lingerie but passes on the ribbons and bows, thank you very much. Calvin Klein will do wonders for him. Stick with smooth fibers in basic colors. Steer clear of prints. Refer to the Practical style in chapter two.

SWEET & INNOCENT GUY

When some men see white cotton panties, it's Game Over. For others, it's a reason to score. Some men *love* the demure, covered-up, innocent look. You can start with white cotton boyshorts and a tank top, or a light-colored babydoll. Knee socks are a plus. Refer to the Romantic/Sweet and Practical styles in chapter two.

True Lingerie Story:

For Sweet & Innocent Guy

My white cotton tap pants were never meant to be sexy; they were purchased purely for comfort. However, my live-in boyfriend (now husband) ignored my sexy, lacy, colorful thongs but always became very attentive and frisky when the tap pants made an appearance. I found this ironic and annoying as I usually had to muster up the nerve to prance around in my carefully selected thong. The thong never caught his eye like the white cotton tap pants. I kept them for a whole decade.

—*Geri W.*, 32DD

TACTILE GUY

Does your man pet you when you're wearing something silky? Does he comment on how good you feel? Does he pout when you wear rough lace? Meet Tactile Guy. He's into how things feel rather than how they look. Simple cuts, such as a basic silk chemise or a satin bra and panty set, will make him crazy with desire. He literally won't be able to keep his hands off you! Look for simple, color-blocked pieces that are classic and silky. Stay away from lace and frills. Refer to Practical style in chapter two, but ditch the cotton. Stay with silk and satin.

VISUAL GUY

Unless they're vision impaired, the majority of men fall into this category. Picture seduction scenes in French movies. Think exquisite lace, shiny black satin, red velvet trim and jewel tone silk gowns. This man is easy to please as long as your lingerie matches and is color coordinated. You can wear anything black, sheer or silky and, rest assured, he will love it. True red or deep-colored lipstick is a must. Refer to the Sophisticated/Chic style in chapter two.

COSTUME GUY

Does he want to be the naughty boss to your secretary, the speeding car driver to your saucy policewoman? Some men like variety in their lives. Spice it up if you're game. If wearing a wig and a French maid's uniform isn't your idea of a good time, try to think of it as playing a role and polishing your theatrical skills. Dress up can be fun! (Especially if you're in a long-term relationship and could stand to stir things up.) Shirley of Hollywood makes a fantastic line of costumes and wigs. Leg Avenue has an amazing array of ultrasexy and creative costumes and legwear.

KINKY GUY

Has he been a very bad boy? Are you supposed to teach him a lesson? Then get out your checklist: riding crop, feather tickler, handcuffs, blindfold. If these items are ringing any bells, you have yourself one kinky man! Relax, tons of men like a little fantasy in their sex lives. There's nothing wrong with some play in your

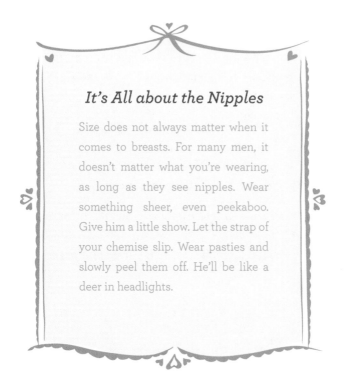

It's All about the Nipples

Size does not always matter when it comes to breasts. For many men, it doesn't matter what you're wearing, as long as they see nipples. Wear something sheer, even peekaboo. Give him a little show. Let the strap of your chemise slip. Wear pasties and slowly peel them off. He'll be like a deer in headlights.

foreplay. If you're a little panicked about the thought of wearing vinyl and leather, don't be. There are plenty of classy kinky options out there. We particularly like Kiki De Montparnasse of New York, where you can find extremely well-made and beautiful lingerie that is still, well, kinky. Refer to the Sexy Seductress section in chapter two.

Seduction Scenarios

Now that you have a better idea about the style of lingerie you should acquire, let the games begin! If you need a hot bath, massage or cocktail to put you in the mood, start there. After all, friskiness is contagious....

Of course, there are limitless applications of lingerie in the bedroom. But here are a few fun ideas to whet your sexual appetite and incorporate your new lingerie into the boudoir.

We rated the following scenarios based on their boldness. If you are a newbie to lingerie—or have a new love—start with Tame. If you want to heat things up, move into Daring or Audacious.

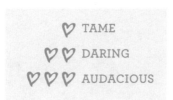

♡ TAME

♡ ♡ DARING

♡ ♡ ♡ AUDACIOUS

♡ ROMANTIC SURPRISE

Be ready in the bedroom when he comes home. Leave a trail of clothing: skirt, blouse, slip and shoes. Turn up the romance with dimmed lights; put scarves over lamp shades to soften the light. Or turn off the lights completely and place candles strategically around the room. Strike a pose or lie seductively on the bed.

True Lingerie Story:

Ho, Ho, Ho

My husband is a lingerie snob. He only likes matching sets; and when I say matching, I mean the same brand and style bra and panty set. One Christmas I received a silly red-and-white Santa outfit, with bells on it, from a girlfriend. Not much to it, just a little tie-side thong and two triangle-shaped cups that tied in the back. It was probably the cheapest lingerie I owned. I put it on and paraded around the room, jingling all the way, for my husband. He absolutely flipped out! He could not keep his hands off me. He told me (several times) later that the outfit was his favorite. You never know what your man might like!

—*Dejha A.*, 36D

♡ WAKE-UP CALL

Too tired for sex at night? Sometimes the thought of dressing up is too exhausting to think about after a long day. Instead, give him a wake-up booty call with a cup of coffee and you in something eye-opening. We suggest a naughty sheer number that leaves nothing to the imagination.

♡ PRE-DATE FLIRT

Encourage him to get off work a little early by sending a picture to his phone of you getting ready for the evening in your date lingerie. Hooray for camera phones!

♡ ♡ CELLULITE CAMOUFLAGE

Most of us have some areas of our bodies we would like to camouflage. Fishnet is the ultimate way to turn flab into fab. Two words: fishnet bodystocking. Is it trashy? Yes. Will you feel a little whorish wearing it? Maybe. Will he die and go to porn-star heaven? Absolutely!

♡ ♡ COME ON, VOGUE

Do not dress up just to run and hide under the covers. Show it off. Not sure how to strike a pose in your lingerie? Start by doing something casual in it. After changing into your sassy number, enter the room and light some candles. Close the blinds. Casually bend over to adjust your ankle strap. Take your time getting to him. He will be crazy with desire when you finally move his way.

♡ ♡ GAMBLIN' MAN

Switch things up by challenging your man to a game of strip poker. Strategically layer your lingerie so each revealing piece drives him more and more crazy. Let him win—you want to make sure you lose your shirt!

♡ ♡ ONE-NIGHT STAND

Make a date to meet him at a swanky hotel bar. (Book a room in advance.) Wear a provocative outfit and titillating lingerie. Pretend you're meeting for the first time. Flirt. Invite him up to your room.

♡ ♡ ♡ FLASHER

The trench coat trick may be cliché, but men are always pleasantly surprised—to say the least—by this tactic. Put on your sexy ensemble and top with a trench coat. Tell him you'll pick him up from work. Let him drive. Flash him some fishnet, a garter or a hint of décolletage. Repeat at stoplights. Drive home safely.

♡ ♡ ♡ VINTAGE BURLESQUE

If you and your partner share a flair for bygone days, surprise him with a private burlesque show! Buy some pasties and frilly knickers and layer with a slip for an old-school peep show. Not sure how to burlesque? Rent a video, take a class or attend a live show to get you in the mood for the curtain call.

♡ ♡ ♡ BIRTHDAY SUIT

Instead of popping out of a cake on his next birthday, bake him a cake and deliver it with a strip tease. Finish off by feeding him a piece of cake in the buff. Be creative with the frosting!

♡ ♡ ♡ ALL TIED UP

Kinky? Yes! That's the point. And the old "tie me to the bed" trick never fails. Take a scarf or specialty cuffs (available at any adult store) and secure your man's hands to the bed. Not all beds accommodate this sort of thing, so be creative. Slowly strip down to your underwear and tease him with your body. The Kinky Guy will appreciate some feathers or other accoutrements. Blindfold is optional.

If love is blind,
why is lingerie so popular?

- ANONYMOUS

CHAPTER 7

Bridal Lingerie

FROM WEDDING AISLE TO HONEYMOON SUITE

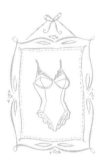

You met a wonderful man. You found the perfect dress. Now comes the hard part: finding the best lingerie for underneath that gorgeous gown. Bridal lingerie should not be an afterthought. After all, the foundations are going to make everything better from fit to comfort, if you choose wisely. And the honeymoon? Plan ahead and you'll blow him away with a trousseau of lingerie from sweet to sex-bomb.

Wedding Day Lingerie

First and foremost, take the pressure off yourself. Many brides try to find the most beautifully breathtaking lingerie that also sucks in, lifts up and generally perfects the body. It does not exist. Beauty and function do not always cooperate when it comes to wedding-day lingerie. It's most important to pick undergarments that make your dress—and you—look amazing. They should make you feel supported, confident and comfortable. Remember, you can change your lingerie between the reception and your first night of marital bliss.

Finding the best-fitting bra or bustier for your wedding gown depends on the gown itself. Its structure, fabric and cut will dictate what you need to wear underneath it. Your best bet is bringing your dress with you when you try on the foundations. We suggest visiting lingerie boutiques, bridal shops or department stores that have experienced staff who are knowledgeable about bridal lingerie. Picking out a pretty bra and panty is one thing; coming up with the right undergarments for a wedding dress is an entirely different matter.

Once you have purchased your lingerie, bring it to your first gown fitting with your tailor. She can then work with your foundations to alter your dress so they go undetected and do their jobs. In some cases, you may even want to consult her before buying your foundations for advice on tricky styles such as backless or deep plunge. The point is to plan ahead and avoid a bridezilla meltdown at the eleventh hour.

Dress Style Considerations

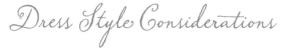

HALTER DRESS

Choose a convertible bra that transforms into a halter or choose to go strapless. If the dress has a plunging back, you can buy a special waist belt that turns your halter bra into a very low-back version that straps around your waist. If you need to go without straps and don't feel comfortable in a strapless bra, choose a bustier without straps.

STRAPLESS DRESS

Select a strapless variety of bustier or bra. If the dress has a low-cut back, look for a long-line, low-back bustier. Small-breasted women may consider having cups sewed into the dress or going sans bra.

SILK DRESS OR
VERY THIN MATERIAL THAT SHOWS EVERYTHING

Buy a smooth, internally boned bustier; we like Le Mystère and Felina. Wear control-top pantyhose or a support short pulled over the bottom seam of the bustier to erase any lines. For dresses with straps, you can invest in a one-piece bodysuit that creates a smoother silhouette. If you're in terrific shape, you might want to go commando and opt for a microfiber bra or discreet nipple covers to protect against air-conditioned reception halls.

Special Tips for Brides

If you wear larger than a DD/E cup and absolutely fall in love with a strapless or backless dress, consider adding straps or having cups and support sewed into the dress. Ask your tailor for a creative solution!

You can find several varieties of stick-on bras for truly backless gowns. While most will stay on, keep things smooth and prevent your nipples from showing, these bras are not going to offer as much support as traditional ones will. If you wear larger than a C cup, you may want to reconsider the style.

If you have never worn a garter belt in your life, do not choose your wedding day to experiment! Practice beforehand to see if you like it; they can be uncomfortable. Save the garter belt for your groom in your room instead.

CORSET-STYLE DRESS

Under this type of dress, everything works. Romantic bridal sets, ruffles and lace, anything goes! If your dress has internal support or boning you can consider going without a bra entirely. Sometimes the least complicated answer is the best one.

True Lingerie Story:

How my Garter Belt got me engaged

After dating my boyfriend for three months, I made a reservation at a local, downtown hotel to celebrate his birthday and New Year's Eve. That night I dressed up special for him with all the bells and whistles, including a garter belt and thigh highs. We were engaged within a month. I like to joke that my garter belt got me engaged. My husband still talks about that night!

—Kim D., 34C

GARTER TOSS

While some couples forgo the tradition of the garter toss, it is still a popular custom that adds a little titillating fun to the reception. There are several garter styles available, from traditional white lace to racy leopard print or colored silk. Choose one that fits your personality, and then let your groom toss it away. If you can't bear to part with it, wear two of them: one for keeps and one to toss.

Honeymoon Lingerie

Now comes the fun part: shopping for your honeymoon lingerie. There are no rules about how much lingerie you should bring or what type. Some say one new outfit per night is expected. Some insist a matching peignoir set is the only way to go, while others think that's passé. What's a girl to do?

Have fun and don't take it all too seriously! The whole point of choosing your honeymoon lingerie collection is to enjoy yourself and be excited that you'll be surprising your groom with outfits that get him excited. Think of this as an excellent opportunity to fill your drawers with romantic and sexy pieces when you return home.

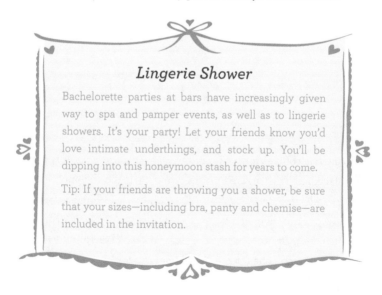

Lingerie Shower

Bachelorette parties at bars have increasingly given way to spa and pamper events, as well as to lingerie showers. It's your party! Let your friends know you'd love intimate underthings, and stock up. You'll be dipping into this honeymoon stash for years to come.

Tip: If your friends are throwing you a shower, be sure that your sizes—including bra, panty and chemise—are included in the invitation.

SUGGESTED PIECES

Whether you spend countless nights in the Bahamas or a luxury weekend in a nearby city, make it a memorable stay—between the sheets. The following is a suggested list of items to bring that will sear the occasion into his memory. Wear these pieces during your honeymoon and beyond. They'll bring back sweet and sexy memories.

TRADITIONAL WEDDING-NIGHT SET

It may be cliché, but most brides dream of being awash in white lace on their first night of married bliss. Don't deny your inner virgin. Go for it! Choose a slinky silk chemise with a matching robe, a hot demi bra with matching panty and garter belt, or anything white and lacy.

PRACTICAL LIGHTWEIGHT ROBE OR WRAP

You'll find this an imperative piece. You will be nude a lot—surprise!—but will still need to cover up occasionally, whether it's for the maid, room service or a midnight stroll to the beach. Look for fabrics like nylon or modal, which won't wrinkle when packed in your suitcase or crumpled in a ball on the side of the bed.

SEXY NIGHTGOWN OR CHEMISE

Simple and elegant. Choose black or vibrantly colored, sheer or lacy. You want to leave just a little bit to the imagination. Very little. This is an especially good choice after a few nights of eating and drinking too much when you still want to feel confident and look ravishing.

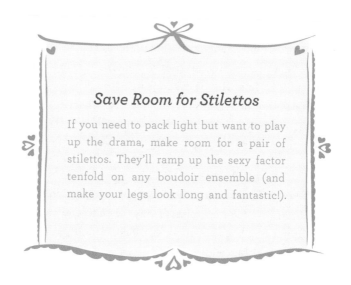

Save Room for Stilettos

If you need to pack light but want to play up the drama, make room for a pair of stilettos. They'll ramp up the sexy factor tenfold on any boudoir ensemble (and make your legs look long and fantastic!).

WILD SOMETHING

Step outside your comfort zone and buy something that is completely outlandish. Go for the whole shebang—think ultraracy, bawdy or kinky. Try a corset or merry widow with matching panty and thigh highs, or something exotic with feathers or tassels. Anything with animal prints is perfect. Pasties or a fishnet bodysuit are sure to fuel the fires of desire. The point is to dress in something utterly unexpected. Smiles and giggles are acceptable with this attire, from both you and your groom.

COMFY SLEEP SET

Consider a soft camisole and short set or a cute matching tank and cropped pants ensemble. After a day at the beach, nothing feels more refreshing on your skin than soft, cool cotton, rayon or modal (and lots of aloe vera). Bring extras sets if you're away more than a few days.

FLIRTY LACE BRA AND PANTY SET

If you already chose a traditional white or ivory set for your wedding night, think about something more fun and colorful. You can keep this ensemble and use it later as your date-night bra and panty set (for when you have a special "date"—with your husband, of course).

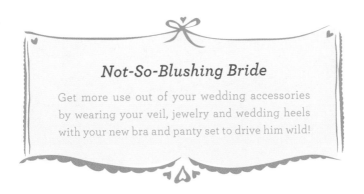

Not-So-Blushing Bride

Get more use out of your wedding accessories by wearing your veil, jewelry and wedding heels with your new bra and panty set to drive him wild!

*I never wear stockings
or underclothes because
I think it is important
to breathe freely.*

- MARILYN MONROE

CHAPTER 8

Lingerie Longevity

CARE AND STORAGE OF YOUR INTIMATES

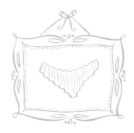

Now that you have a chest full of flattering apparel and sexy underthings, you'll want to ensure your lingerie's longevity. The two most important factors in caring for your delicates are washing and storage. First, it's imperative to launder your bras and panties properly. After all, they are the closest thing to you, taking on your body oils and sweat more than your clothing. Next important is preservation. Poor storage habits lead to misshaped or, even worse, lost lingerie. If you can't find it, you can't enjoy it! So let's get busy and do the wash first.

Washing Your Bras:
The Eternal Dilemma

How often should you wash a bra? Some manufacturers recommend doing so after every time you wear it. We all know that's just not practical! If you are out dancing all night in it, however, by all means wash it. We believe bras should be washed according to how much you wear them. Our rule of thumb is up to four "gentle wears" (no sweating or excessive activity) before sending your bra to the laundry room. If you wear it once a week, wash it once a month. If you wear it every day, wash it at least once a week. We do, although, recommend a day of rest for your overworked bras, to let the fibers regain their elasticity. Try not to wear the same bra more than two days in a row.

Wash Day Wisdom

Always read care tags attached to each garment. This should be a no-brainer, but we've all ignored these informative little labels. The results are shrunken panties, deformed bras and irreparable messes.

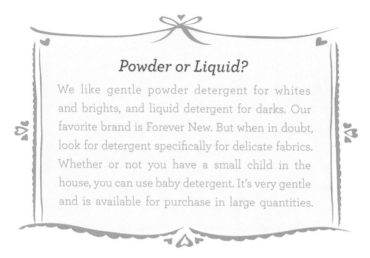

Powder or Liquid?

We like gentle powder detergent for whites and brights, and liquid detergent for darks. Our favorite brand is Forever New. But when in doubt, look for detergent specifically for delicate fabrics. Whether or not you have a small child in the house, you can use baby detergent. It's very gentle and is available for purchase in large quantities.

HAND WASH

We strongly suggest you hand wash your lingerie. Yes, this can be a boring process—unless you make it fun! Put on your favorite music and thumb through magazines while your panties soak. Or put on your Bluetooth headset and call your boyfriend while you wash his favorite bra and panty set.

STEP 1.   Add a small amount of gentle detergent to your sink and fill with lukewarm water.

STEP 2.   Separate your lights from your darks, and wash a couple items of similar color at the same time. Soak them for a minute or two in the sink.

STEP 3.   Rinse with cool water.

STEP 4.   Gently squeeze any excess water from the items. Line dry or lie flat on a towel.

MACHINE WASH

Hand washing is ideal, but if you must machine wash, follow these tips. If you have a washing machine with an agitator in the middle, we suggest you do not wash your bras in it. It's too abrasive on delicates and can mangle underwire bras beyond recognition. (Ever have an underwire pop out of your bra?) Newer front-load models have a hand-wash cycle that won't manhandle most bras. Nevertheless, always use a lingerie laundry bag. This mesh or lace bag zips up and protects delicate items from getting damaged. You can find one at any lingerie boutique and most major department stores in the intimate-apparel department.

STEP 1. Put any lacy or especially delicate items in a lingerie laundry bag. If washing your bras, hook them before you put them in, to avoid snagging other items. Zip the bag and place it in your washing machine. Add any other items that don't require the extra protection, such as a modal chemise or polyester pajamas.

STEP 2. Add your delicate detergent and set the temperature to warm or cold, with cool rinse. Use the hand-wash cycle if available; otherwise, choose the delicate setting.

STEP 3. When the cycle is done, remove your delicate items from the bag and lay them flat on a towel or line dry.

STEP 4. Though we do not recommend it (more details follow), you may put some items (never bras) in the dryer. This would include pieces fabricated from cotton or some synthetics per the manufacturer instructions. Promptly remove any items from the dryer to avoid wrinkles.

Special Attention for Underpants

Because of where your panties have been, your inclination may be to wash them in scalding water. Read our pouty, rouged lips: Don't do it. You'll ruin them. Our method is to first run very warm water over the crotch for about thirty seconds. Next, lightly scrub this area by rubbing the fabric together. Then, soak for a couple of minutes. Give your underpants one or two rinses to get the soap out, and lie flat or line dry.

THE DRYER IS THE DEVIL

Have you ever pulled a pair of panties out of the dryer that looked like something from a low-budget horror film? Those white or black "worms" are the result of the devilish dryer breaking down and melting the elastic. Never, ever put your bras or delicate panties in the dryer. It shortens their life span.

True Lingerie Story:

Blowing in the Wind

I had a small clothesline in my backyard where I would hang my unmentionables during good weather after hand washing them. One day when I was out, my husband and his buddy came back from a golf game. They went out on the patio to have a beer. There hung all my black lacy underwear, bras and teddies. The buddy said, "Those slutty panties can't be your wife's!" My husband just smiled and left them hanging.

—Kathy S., 34D

FABRIC CARE

All fabrics are not created equal—and should not be washed the same way. While we encourage you to follow the manufacturer's instructions on the garment tag, we have some suggestions for specific fabrics.

COTTON—Machine wash in cold, warm or hot water, on permanent press or delicate cycle. Read tags to be sure, but most cotton is okay to put in the dryer on medium heat.

LINEN—Machine wash on delicate cycle, in cool to lukewarm water, or hand wash. Air dry and press with an iron. This fabric can also be dry-cleaned.

NYLON—Hand wash in cool water and air dry.

POLYESTER AND OTHER SYNTHETICS—Machine wash cold, with like colors, on delicate cycle. Air dry or use low heat setting on the dryer.

RAYON, MODAL, VISCOSE AND FABRICS MADE FROM WOOD OR BAMBOO FIBERS—In cold water, machine wash on delicate cycle, or hand wash. Air dry, or can also be dry-cleaned.

SILK—Hand wash in cool water with a liquid detergent for delicates. Do not rub or squeeze silk when it's wet, as the fibers are weaker at that time. Place garment between two towels to gently press dry. Iron when damp. Silk can also be dry-cleaned.

WOOL AND CASHMERE—Dry-cleaning is recommended. If you hand wash, use a detergent for wool or delicates and soak for up to five minutes in lukewarm water. Squeeze gently, rinse and lay flat to dry.

Organizing Your Lingerie

How many times have you spent valuable minutes in the morning digging in your drawer for a particular pair of panties? Our underwear is the first thing we reach for when getting dressed. Shouldn't it be sorted out and easy to select? You not only want to save time, but also extend your lingerie's shelf life. Don't get your panties in a twist by jamming them into drawers! Likewise, avoid crushed bra cups with proper storage.

First you need to assess your space. Do you have a large dresser and cramped closet, or a walk-in closet with minimal drawer space? Do you own a lingerie chest or have an extra closet to use? Keep in mind that you use your bras and panties every day, so easy access should be a top priority. If you need to, get creative with your space constraints.

GENERAL ORGANIZATION

Whether you use dresser drawers, a lingerie chest or your closet, organizing by color and/or style makes life easier.

BY COLOR

If you tend to match your lingerie to your outfits, organize by color.

Panties:

- Black
- Green, blue and purple
- Nude and nude prints
- Print, floral and striped
- Red, orange and yellow

Bras:

- Black
- Colored
- Nude and white

BY STYLE

Panties:

- Boyshorts, bikinis and other fuller-coverage styles
- Thongs

Bras:

- Bra and panty sets
- Everyday bras
- Special/sexy bras

IN DRESSER DRAWERS

A popular way of organizing panties and bras is to assign panties to one drawer and bras to another. Here's how to do it.

Panties: Organize your panties to make daily selection easy. You can either purchase a drawer organizer with several cubbies for each individual pair, or create two sections, one for thongs and one for bikinis and boyshorts. You may also have multi-sections to organize by color or style. Simply fold your panties into a tidy square and store them in their section, or roll the panties into a neat cylinder and tuck them into their individual cubbies.

Bras: Bras should be hooked so they don't catch on other items. If you have little space, you can fold your bras in half and store them in a drawer. Fold one cup into another on contour bras so the cups don't crease. Organize by color or style.

IN THE CLOSET

Sleepwear, slips, camisoles and robes should hang in your closet. You can use traditional hangers or choose some pretty, padded ones, which are gentle on your silk and knitwear. If you must store these items in your dresser, be warned: they tend to get lost in the back of drawers and wrinkled beyond recognition. Give them their own full drawer for easy selection.

Panties, etc.: If you have ample closet space, create a little miniboutique for yourself! Purchase four bins or baskets and arrange them on a shelf or in a cubby. We do not recommend wicker ones unless they are lined; they can snag your delicates.

> BIN 1: Thongs
> BIN 2: Full-coverage panties (bikinis, boyshorts, etc.)
> BIN 3: Hosiery and socks
> BIN 4: Shapewear and sports bras

Bras: Unless you have a closet built specifically with space for hanging your bras, don't hang them with your clothes; they will certainly get lost if you do. You can find hosiery- and shoe-storage bags, with clear plastic window sections, that can work for small sizes of underwire cups and soft bras. Simply hook, fold and insert a bra into each pocket. We like this solution because you can easily identify your bras at a moment's glance! If you have only a limited number of bras, you may be able to keep them in a bin in your closet (see advice on panties above). Make sure to hook your bras when storing and ensure the cups are not misshapen or squished.

IN A LINGERIE CHEST

If you have a full dresser and closet, and are straining to find room for your underthings, invest in a lingerie chest! This furnishing is a tall tower of single-wide drawers. A lingerie chest typically has six drawers but can have more or fewer. It comes in different styles, from traditional to contemporary, so it's easy to find something that will match your decor. Here are some ideas on what to put in each drawer.

- Basic everyday bras
- Bra and panty sets (finally store them together!)
- Hosiery
- Knee highs and socks
- Panties, by color
  (all black in one drawer and colors in another)
- Panties, by style
- Shapewear
- Soft bras and/or sports bras

SOME CREATIVE SOLUTIONS

Run out of room in your room? Consider putting your lingerie chest in your closet. You can stack shoe boxes or handbags on top of it.

Stackable bins with pullout drawers can go in your closet underneath hanging blouses or short skirts. Fill them with panties, socks, hosiery or bras.

Hooks on the inside of your closet doors can hold an array of everyday bras.

Have a walk-in closet? Store special pieces in bins on top shelves; keep a small step stool inside to reach them easily.

STORING FOR LATER USE

Storage may be the answer if you have an extensive collection of lingerie; have fluctuated sizes and want to keep pieces for future ups and downs; or are short on space. Here are some storage solutions.

Bras: See-through, plastic storage containers or canvas containers with clear viewing windows are the best ways to store your bras. You can find shoe box–size clear bins with lids and can store several bras in each container. These usually fit snugly in your closet or under your bed. Clear storage is preferable because you can see what is in each bin without sorting through each one when you need something.

Bra and panty sets: These can be stored the same way, keeping individual sets in each container. If you have several different sizes, appropriately mark the outside of each bin.

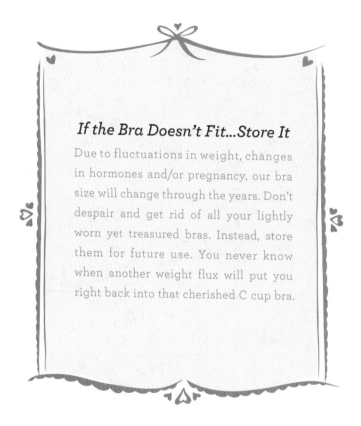

If the Bra Doesn't Fit...Store It

Due to fluctuations in weight, changes in hormones and/or pregnancy, our bra size will change through the years. Don't despair and get rid of all your lightly worn yet treasured bras. Instead, store them for future use. You never know when another weight flux will put you right back into that cherished C cup bra.

Shop Talk

TIPS, TRICKS AND WHERE TO GO

Time to shop! We've got some quick tips for you and some of our favorite places to frequent, both brick and mortar and online.

Shopping Tips

MAKE TIME

Purchasing lingerie you love requires more than a snap decision. Try not to do it on a hurried lunch hour when shops are busy. You'll leave frustrated and disheveled. Schedule a block of time when you can shop at a leisurely pace and try on items without rushing. Have an idea of what you need and want. Keep a mental or paper list.

BE OPEN TO SUGGESTIONS

Don't just run to that three-for panty rounder at the department store. New styles come out every season and sometimes we just get in a buying rut. Ask for advice and assistance. Experienced salespeople who know their products can introduce new items and help you think outside the box. They can recommend brands that fit your body type.

BECOME FAMILIAR WITH SHOPS AND BRANDS

Shops often tout their brands and become known for the designers they carry. Get to know both and you'll be able to gauge price range and style. One word of warning: Don't get into a brand rut! You'll miss some beautiful and exciting pieces from other designers.

SHOP BY STYLE

Shop with your favorite styles in mind: Sporty, Sophisticated, Sweet & Innocent, etc. It's efficient and will help keep you on track.

APPLY WHAT YOU'VE LEARNED

Maybe your apple-shaped body has always worn two-piece jammie sets. Try a chemise and feel like a new woman.

THINK ABOUT YOUR WARDROBE

Are you missing a black slip? A plunge bra? Did you just buy a new dress that requires patterned hosiery? Check your closet before you shop.

TAKE TIME TO MAKE A DECISION

Sometimes you immediately know if something looks smashing or if you absolutely love it. Then buy it! If you're unsure (does it look good, do you need it, does if fill a hole in your lingerie drawer...), have the clerk hold your selection. Go have a latte and deliberate. It will save you time (taking things back) and money (no-return policies).

WATCH FOR SALES

A sale is a great time to try a new brand or style to see how you like it, pick up multiple panties in shades to match your bras and buy shapewear.

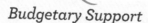

Budgetary Support

We can't stress enough how important it is to search out a reliable department store or boutique where you can be fit for a bra. However, once you know your size, you can find some bargains on brassieres other places.

- Check out Ross, Marshalls, T.J. Maxx, Nordstrom Rack, Filene's Basement and any other discount stores that carry off-price designer brands. Often you can score department store brands discounted more than 50 percent.

- Websites which offer a variety of brands are great places for basics such as T-shirt bras by Maidenform and Vanity Fair. These bras cost less than thirty dollars, feel comfortable and create a great shape under clothing.

- Check out the fun, flirty bras at Target for less than twenty dollars! We like the Gilligan & O'Malley brand for its youthful, flirty styles and prints.

- Sign up on the mailing lists of your favorite lingerie shops for advance notification of sales.

- Join the e-mail lists on Web sites. There are almost always online specials.

- Buy in bulk. Shops will often have specials on panties when you buy several. Stock up on your favorite styles.

Stores

Our list is far from exhaustive, but we've provided some lovely places for you to start. We've noted which brick-and-mortar stores also sell online.

CALIFORNIA

AGENT PROVOCATEUR
7961 MELROSE AVENUE
LOS ANGELES, CA 90046
323-653-0229
PLUS ADDITIONAL LOCATIONS
WWW.AGENTPROVOCATEUR.COM
(SELLS ONLINE)

Provocative is the operative word here. This United Kingdom-based purveyor of pricey lingerie offers lots of frilly and lacy ensembles— under names such as Cherry, Fanny and Natasha—and a wide variety of garter belts and stockings. There are also stores in New York, Las Vegas and Miami.

EAST 13TH
356 E. COLORADO BOULEVARD
PASADENA, CA 91101
626-795-9386
PLUS ADDITIONAL LOCATION
WWW.EAST13.COM
(SELLS ONLINE)

You won't find anything pink in this male-friendly shop, but you will find mid- to high-end glamorous lines such as Marlies Dekkers and Huit. The store offers bra fitting, free deliveries and hard-to-find sizes from 28AA to 52K. Try your selection in a sultry purple, ivory and black dressing room with mirrored ceilings, comfy seating and plush pillows. Your partner is welcome inside to check the fit.

FAIRE FROU FROU
13017A VENTURA BOULEVARD
STUDIO CITY, CA 91604
818-783-4970
WWW.FAIREFROUFROU.COM
(SELLS ONLINE)

This shop specializes in on-trend lingerie and intimate apparel that doubles as apparel. The bright Parisian-style boutique offers distinctively high-end brands such as Carine Gilson Lingerie Couture, Damaris, and Vannina Vesperini. Color-coordinated displays make for easy shopping.

FREDERICK'S OF HOLLYWOOD
6751 HOLLYWOOD BOULEVARD
HOLLYWOOD, CA 90028
323-957-5953
PLUS ADDITIONAL LOCATIONS
WWW.FREDERICKS.COM
(SELLS ONLINE)

Founder Frederick Mellinger launched his legendary lingerie line in 1946. Since then, the company has branched out from Tinseltown to Worcester. This lingerie wonderland is packed with panties from $1.99, to corsets and costumes for every fantasy.

LISA NORMAN LINGERIE, ETC.
1134 MONTANA AVENUE
SANTA MONICA, CA 90403
310-451-2026
877-547-2667
WWW.LISANORMAN.COM

Lisa Norman specializes in beautiful European lingerie with an emphasis on natural fibers and fantastic fit. In that sense, this 30-year-old shop is perfect for the low-maintenance minimalist who wants quality foundations. Clients appreciate exemplary assistance from an experienced staff.

Lula Lu

212 E. THIRD AVENUE
SAN MATEO, CA 94401
650-348-8858
WWW.LULALU.COM
(SELLS ONLINE)

Pert and petite girls will love Ellen Shing's lingerie shop. She caters to women who wear AA and A cups and is a master fitter for these small-busted ladies. The emphasis is on extra small and small sizes, but stock runs up to C cups and larger, too. You'll find it all, from bras to corsets, and brands including Bodas, Princesse tam.tam, and Shing's own Lula Lu line.

Lulu's

300 MANHATTAN BEACH BOULEVARD
MANHATTAN BEACH, CA 90266
310-798-4577
WWW.LULUSMB.COM

Fuel your female passions at this vintage-inspired shop filled with shoes, jewelry, chocolates, candles and, of course, lingerie. The store carries everything from basic to fancy in classic romantic colors: black, ivory, white, soft pink and leopard prints. Favorites include La Perla, Cosabella, Skin Lingerie, and Wendy Glez. The gift wrap is gorgeous.

My Boudoir Lingerie

2029 FILLMORE STREET
SAN FRANCISCO, CA 94115
415-346-1502
WWW.MYBOUDOIR.NET

Owner Geraldine Moreno Nuval knows the power of lingerie and seeks out styles for women who want something different and who aren't afraid of color. She carries lines such as Marlies Dekkers, I.D. Sarrieri, and Falke. The bohemian boudoir vibe sets the mood for selecting sexy pieces for the boudoir portraits offered by the store. Don't forget to ask about custom-made corsets.

TOUJOURS LINGERIE
2484 SACRAMENTO STREET
SAN FRANCISCO, CA 94115
415-346-3988
888-621-9397
WWW.TOUJOURSLINGERIE.COM

Loyal customers have frequented this pretty, peach-and-ivory, just-bigger-than-a-walk-in-closet-size shop for more than twenty-two years. Choose from carefully curated, sophisticated styles in brands such as Lise Charmel, Nina Ricci, and Prima Donna. Luxurious Pluto sleepwear is available as well.

TRASHY LINGERIE
402 N. LA CIENEGA BOULEVARD
LOS ANGELES, CA 90048
310-652-4543
WWW.TRASHY.COM
(SELLS ONLINE)

Here it's costumes galore, reform-school girls to pussycats; every kind of hosiery, from butt baring hose to red fishnets; fingerless vinyl gloves; pasties; cupless bras; an abundance of bows; see-through somethings.... Well, you get the picture. You can't miss the big pink building—it's been there for thirty-five years.

COLORADO

SOL
248 DETROIT STREET
DENVER, CO 80206
800-466-1356
WWW.SOLLINGERIE.COM
(SELLS ONLINE)

Fit is at the top of the list at this warm and inviting Tuscan-vibe boutique complete with a fish-filled fountain. European lingerie includes brands from Marie Jo, Andres Sarda, and Aubade. Ask about personal shopping services for your wedding night. The staff is also happy to help a man select something special for his girl.

FLORIDA

COSABELLA FLAGSHIP BOUTIQUE
760 OCEAN DRIVE, #7
MIAMI BEACH, FL 33139
888-534-4731
WWW.COSABELLA.COM

The flagship U.S. shop has it all from this favored Italian-made line famous for its feminine thong and penchant for color. Choose from bra and panty sets, camis, chemises, loungewear, swimwear and more.

UNDERWRAPS
610 E. LAS OLAS BOULEVARD
FORT LAUDERDALE, FL 33301
954-522-2227

Known for professional customer service, meticulous fitting techniques and a great mix of essentials, this award-winning lingerie boutique is filled with old-world charm and fashion-forward European lingerie. Love Le Mystère? Underwraps carries the full line.

GEORGIA

Intimacy

3500 Peachtree Road N.E.
Phipps Plaza
Atlanta, GA 30326
404-261-9333
Plus additional locations
www.myintimacy.com

Susan Nethero, owner of this Atlanta-based chain, trained under June Kenton, bra fitter for the queen of England. Her pedigree also extends to fitting Oprah. Bra fitting here is radically different. There is no tape measure; the method is considered holistic, taking a woman's contours into account. More than 80 percent of the brands Intimacy carries are European and the variety is impressive, with options from A to K cups, bands from 32 to 48, and dozens of styles. Check online for a store near (or coming soon) to you.

Oh! Fine Lingerie

178 Peachtree Hills Avenue
Atlanta, GA 30305
404-949-9901
www.ohfinelingerie.com

Owner Sandy Thigpen is fond of admonishing women to "wear it for him...before he buys it for her." And she has plenty of pieces to choose from in her European-style shop. Thigpen can even have your selection customized. Brides will find the best here from Vera Wang, Claire Pettibone, and Simone Pérèle. Special orders are part of the shop's excellent service.

ILLINOIS

G. BOUTIQUE
2131 N. DAMEN AVENUE
CHICAGO, IL 60647
773-235-1234
WWW.BOUTIQUEG.COM
(SELLS ONLINE)

Pretty in pink, this shop strives to create a comfortable environment for women to gather in. G Boutique carries lines such as Cosabella, Hanky Panky, Simone Pérèle, and Huit. Need a few pointers on parading around in your new purchases? The store offers workshops, classes and photo sessions where gals can pose as pinup girls and vogue like burlesque queens.

ISABELLA FINE LINGERIE
840 W. ARMITAGE AVENUE
CHICAGO, IL 60614
773-281-2352
PLUS ADDITIONAL LOCATION
WWW.SHOPISABELLA.COM
(SELLS ONLINE)

This sophisticated, well-organized shop stocks lingerie from basic bras to sexy little numbers from Le Mystère, Cosabella, Honeydew, Huit, and La Perla. If you need some extra oomph in your bra or tricks to avert a fashion faux pas, this shop can help. Owner Lauren Armerine (aka the Bra Psychic) has an uncanny knack for guessing bra sizes.

UNDERTHINGS
804 W. WEBSTER AVENUE
CHICAGO, IL 60614
773-472-9291

In business for nearly three decades, Underthings offers clients personal services, consulting, fittings, gifts, lingerie and foundations. You'll find quality brands such as Natori and HANRO. Styles appeal to the young and restless, as well as to those with more classic tastes.

WILDFLOWERS LINGERIE
1407 N. WELLS STREET
CHICAGO, IL 60610
312-654-0482
WWW.SHOPWILDFLOWERS.COM
(SELLS ONLINE)

Inside this old European-style courtyard you'll find a cozy boutique that focuses on service and value over frivolous and flimsy. Fitters work to resolve issues, provide proper fit and suggest underthings appropriate for your personal wardrobe. Favorites here include Simone Pérèle, Huit, Arianne, and Wendy Glez. You'll find great lounge and sleepwear, silk lingerie and pieces for the sophisticated lady. Private appointments for couples are available.

MASSACHUSETTS

FRENCH LESSONS
26 STATE STREET
NEWBURYPORT, MA 01950
978-499-0499
PLUS ADDITIONAL LOCATIONS

This boutique is very much like a Parisian atelier where Colette would have been proud to write her prose. Trained "fitresses" will put you in the right foundations. In fact, they won't let you out the door if your underwear doesn't totally flatter you in your outerwear. Firm believers that you can still be sexy in your forties and beyond, the buyers supply styles that flatter a variety of body types. You'll find a nice selection of shapewear and brands such as Cosabella, Princesse tam.tam, eberjey, and Le Mystère.

MICHIGAN

BON FITTE
206 E. FRONT STREET
TRAVERSE CITY, MI 49684
231-929-8997
WWW.BONFITTEBRASSIERE
BOUTIQUE.COM

The name of this bra-centric shop says it all: Good Fit, en français. It's easy to find—just look for the quaint shop with pretty windows. It's situated in an historical building on the town's main street. Among the mid- to high-range lingerie brands, you'll find Mystique Intimates, Shirley of Hollywood, Hanky Panky, and RubyPink. Bra sizes run from 30 to 56 bands and from A to JJ cups. Bonus: a nice selection of bustiers.

LORI KARBAL
554 N. OLD WOODWARD AVENUE
BIRMINGHAM, MI 48009
248-258-1959
WWW.LORIKARBAL.COM

This sophisticated shabby chic shop with Venetian chandeliers carries a host of accessible lingerie. Choose from lots of pretty pajama sets from Cosabella, Hanky Panky, eberjey, P.J. Salvage, and the übercomfy DreamSacks loungewear. This is also a great place to pick up beauty products such as the heavenly scented Santa Maria Novella soaps.

NEVADA

BLACK SATIN INTIMATES
AT THE WYNN LAS VEGAS
WYNN ESPLANADE
3131 LAS VEGAS BOULEVARD S.
LAS VEGAS, NV 89109
702-770-3450

Celebrate your win at the blackjack table with a little something from this elegant shop, bedecked with dramatic black crystal chandeliers, located inside the Wynn Las Vegas hotel. Choose from luxury lingerie and hot negligees from Marlies Dekkers, Huit, and Vera Wang. Or pick up a new toy from Kiki De Montparnasse. Remember, what happens in Vegas, stays in Vegas.

NEW JERSEY

GEORGIE GIRL BOUTIQUE
105 KINGS HIGHWAY E.
HADDONFIELD, NJ 08033
856-354-4700
WWW.GEORGIEGIRLBOUTIQUE.COM
(SELLS ONLINE)

Jersey girls are lucky indeed to have this well-stocked boutique. The shop is filled with lingerie that runs from fun and flirty to classic and elegant. Brands include Josie Natori, Aubade, Cosabella, and Jonquil. Clients gush about the service (special delivery of packages, phone calls about sales and new merchandise, and personal touches you'd expect from a good girlfriend). Ask about the girl gatherings: in-store pj and lingerie parties.

NEW YORK

AZALEAS
223 E. TENTH STREET
NEW YORK, NY 10003
212-253-5484
800-775-0540
WWW.AZALEASNYC.COM
(SELLS ONLINE)

This very girlish, hot-pink boutique has one rule: everything has to be soft to the touch. It's also a good source for some of the prettiest underwear as outerwear. Styles from CLO, Huit, and Princesse tam.tam are flirty, feminine and colorful. Shopping is simple rather than overwhelming: only one of each item is on display in the uncluttered store.

KIKI DE MONTPARNASSE
79 GREENE STREET
NEW YORK, NY 10012
212-965-8150
PLUS ADDITIONAL LOCATION
WWW.KIKIDM.COM

This shop sets the mood for its wares with a decor that screams SEX. But in an upscale, urban way. The store stocks provocative lingerie for discerning clients who love beautiful things to create steamy fantasies. Unleash the seductress within while you shop for quintessential black lingerie, handcuffs and "instruments of pleasure."

LA PETITE COQUETTE
51 UNIVERSITY PLACE
NEW YORK, NY 10003
212-473-2478
888-473-5799
WWW.THELITTLEFLIRT.COM
(SELLS ONLINE)

Known for bringing out the little flirt in every gal, owner Rebecca Apsan is a walking encyclopedia of lingerie. It's all here in this romantic lingerie emporium: European designs, bustiers, styles for curvaceous women and more brands than you can shake your booty at.

MIXONA
262 MOTT STREET
NEW YORK, NY 10012
646-613-0100
WWW.MIXONA.COM

Classic cuts, lace trimming and silk sleepwear top the list of sensual treats at this Eurocentric lingerie boutique. The shop specializes in brands such as Dolce & Gabbana, Chantal Thomass, Argentovivo, and Mimi Holliday. Check out their affordable namesake label while you're there. Getting hitched? The store hosts bridal showers and bachelorette parties in their private-event salon.

ORCHARD CORSET CENTER
157 ORCHARD STREET
NEW YORK, NY 10002
212-674-0786
WWW.ORCHARDCORSET.COM
(SELLS ONLINE)

This is not your mother's bra shop. It's more like your grandmother's: shapewear for your butt and gut are still called girdles. But it's great for functional foundations, corsets and basics at reasonable prices.

SLEEP
110 N. SIXTH STREET
BROOKLYN, NY 11211
718-384-3211
WWW.SLEEPBROOKLYN.COM
(SELLS ONLINE)

Not surprisingly, this shop is known for its excellent selection of sleepwear. You'll find elegant, natural fibers at this French boudoir–style boutique where the focus is on stellar designers like Stella McCartney. An array of enticing bra and panty sets is also available.

TOWN SHOP
2273 BROADWAY
NEW YORK, NY 10024
212-787-2762
WWW.TOWNSHOP.COM

An institution for more than 120 years, they've served generations, fit thousands of women and sold an untold number of bras. The selection is enormous and ranges from AA to JJ bras, shapewear, sleepwear, hosiery, and panties from thongs to maximum coverage briefs. You'll find brands such as Aubade, Wacoal, Cosabella, Chantelle, Wolford, and Lejaby.

NORTH CAROLINA

I.C. LONDON
1419 EAST BOULEVARD, SUITE F
CHARLOTTE, NC 28203
704-377-7955
PLUS ADDITIONAL LOCATION
WWW.ICLONDON.COM
(SELLS ONLINE)

This very girlie shop is conveniently organized with bras, panties and shapewear on one side and sleepwear and loungewear on the other. They carry 30A to 40KK bra sizes and alter them to boot (for example, cutting a band down from 32 to 30). Check out the organic cotton sleepwear and don't miss the Huit Magic Pulp panties: they add a little junk in the trunk for those dresses that demand a J. Lo rear.

OREGON

JANE'S VANITY
521 S.W. BROADWAY AVENUE
PORTLAND, OR 97205
503-241-3860
WWW.JANESVANITY.COM

There is a true sense of intimacy while buying your intimates in this little jewel box of a shop. Owner Jane Adams searches for the loveliest lingerie and is known for her personalized shopping services. You'll find styles by Andres Sarda, Chantal Thomass, and other European designers.

OH BABY
1811 N.E. BROADWAY STREET
PORTLAND, OR 97232
503-281-7430
PLUS ADDITIONAL LOCATION
WWW.OHBABYLINGERIESHOPS.COM

With two lovely locations to choose from, Portlanders are spoiled by the personal service at these sultry boutiques. These shops carry lines such as Aubade, Huit, and Marlies Dekkers, and pretty silky things from Jonquil. They also cater to brides looking for the perfect dress foundations and honeymoon lingerie. High-end accessories (read: toys) are also available.

SOUTH CAROLINA

BITS OF LACE
302 KING STREET
CHARLESTON, SC 29401
843-577-0999
WWW.BITSOFLACE.COM
(SELLS ONLINE)

Old-world charm pervades this boutique nestled in an historic building with hardwood floors and original crown molding. Women who love high-end lingerie flock to the shop for European brands such as Eres, Celestine, and Conturelle. Appointments are available for bra fittings.

TEXAS

LA MODE LINGERIE
2013D W. GRAY
HOUSTON, TX 77019
713-529-3980
WWW.LAMODELINGERIE.COM

Sleek, modern and decked out in white, this shop has a gallery-like atmosphere and caters to sophisticates. It specializes in French and Italian lines such as Chantelle, Simone Pérèle, and I.D. Sarrieri. Love the bra but the fit isn't quite right? The store offers custom fitting and bra alterations.

UNDERWEAR
916B W. TWELFTH STREET
AUSTIN, TX 78703
512-478-1515
WWW.FETISHAUSTIN.COM

Plainly stated, this Austin shop sells underwear—but the good stuff. The tranquil boudoirlike setting features high-end lingerie such as Kiki De Montparnasse, Wendy Glez, and Princesse tam.tam. Selections are decidedly classic, elegant and sexy. It's a great place for bridal gift shopping, too.

VIRGINIA

TROUSSEAU
306 MAPLE AVENUE W.
VIENNA, VA 22180
703-255-3300
WWW.TROUSSEAULTD.COM

As the name suggests, the focus here is on bridal lingerie, from foundations beneath your wedding gown to sumptuous silk and satin for the wedding night. However, the shop also carries lingerie (albeit beautiful European lines) for the more mundane days of our lives.

WASHINGTON

ANN MARIE LINGERIE
4000 E. MADISON STREET
SEATTLE, WA 98112
206-323-6027

Ladies Who Lunch love this classic lingerie boutique where selections are in tasteful tones of ivory, white, petal-pink and black. Oh, and a bit of leopard print, à la Mrs. Robinson, to spice things up. You'll find lovely negligees and sleepwear from Celeste and Pluto, Dana Pisarra camis as well as bra and panty sets from Huit and Barbara. They also specialize in luscious long silk gowns and offer gorgeous choices for brides-to-be.

BELLEFLEUR LINGERIE BOUTIQUE
720 N. THIRTY-FIFTH STREET
SEATTLE, WA 98103
206-545-0222
WWW.BELLEFLEURLINGERIE.COM

Lively, playful and sexy are among the many types of lingerie options you'll find at Jennifer Carroll's feminine shop. The expert bra fitter has a warm and welcoming manner and puts women at ease as she puts them into the perfect lingerie ensemble to accentuate their positive assets. Her well-trained staff will help you find beautiful items from European and designer lines such as Cosabella, Aubade, Betsey Johnson, and Huit. Ask about in-store lingerie events, after-hours shopping parties, bachelorette parties and bridal showers.

NANCY MEYER FINE LINGERIE
1318 FIFTH AVENUE
SEATTLE, WA 98101
800-605-5098
WWW.NANCYMEYER.COM
(SELLS ONLINE)

Lingerie connoisseurs will find the finest luxury lingerie at this high-end, downtown, European-style boutique. In business for more than twenty-five years, the boutique carries an exemplary collection of what women want: cozy cashmere robes from Daniel Hanson, racy bra and panty sets by Eres and the most sublime lacy pieces by Carine Gilson. If you're looking for a place to splurge on a pair of three-hundred-dollar panties this is it. If you can't make it into the store, a sophisticated online shop awaits.

ZOVO LINGERIE
4612 TWENTY-SIXTH AVENUE N.E.
UNIVERSITY VILLAGE
SEATTLE, WA 98105
206-525-9686
888-525-9686
WWW.ZOVOLINGERIE.COM
(SELLS ONLINE)

Victoria Roberts launched her store with a focus on fitting women in beautiful lingerie and offering a shopping experience in a richly appointed environment. Inspired by southern Spain, the shop features terracotta stucco walls, arches, warm-toned woods, wrought-iron fixtures and velvet-curtained dressing rooms. Women come here for a wide range of bra sizes from brands such as Princesse tam.tam, Prima Donna, Chantelle, and Roberts's own Zovo line of fine cotton panties and loungewear.

WASHINGTON, D.C.

COUP DE FOUDRE LINGERIE
1001 PENNSYLVANIA AVENUE N.W.
WASHINGTON, DC 20004
202-393-0878
WWW.COUPDEFOUDRELINGERIE.COM
(SELLS ONLINE)

The focus here is classy and elegant European lingerie from Chantelle, Simone Pérèle, Huit, Jonquil, Prima Donna, and Cosabella. Saleswomen with French accents lend an air of sophistication to this bright and airy lingerie shop. Expert bra fitters all, they'll also help you with foundations under special dresses and offer personal shopping services for men.

Online

WWW.AGENTPROVOCATEUR.COM
You'll want to engage your wild side with these pieces. Provocative lingerie with lots of garter belt options.

WWW.BARENECESSITIES.COM
Here, you'll find a huge range of brands, from affordable to luxe, and an impressive bra selection, including sports bras that eschew the "uniboob." Sales are ongoing and varied and shipping is inexpensive.

WWW.BEDHEADPJS.COM
This website carries a plethora of prints in classic pj's in quality cottons and flannel. Lots of cute cami sets, robes and loungewear, too.

WWW.BELLAMATERNA.COM
This Seattle-based company uses luxury Italian microfiber in their contemporary and sophisticated lingerie and maternity pieces. Their line is equally comfortable before, during and after pregnancy.

WWW.CATRIONAMACKECHNIE.COM
Focus is on the best lingerie in terms of design, quality and styling. A well-edited selection.

WWW.DESIGNERINTIMATES.COM
Affordable selection of lingerie with an emphasis on Jezebel and Felina brands.

WWW.FIGLEAVES.COM
Lots of everything: more than one hundred brands, with easy shopping by category, style and "what's hot." Generous offerings for full-figured gals.

WWW.FREDERICKSOFHOLLYWOOD.COM
Sexy, sexy. All sorts of peekaboo lingerie from teddies to bustiers. At these low prices, you can go crazy.

WWW.FRESHPAIR.COM
Good for basics. The brands range from Playtex and Maidenform to some choice pieces from Chantelle.

WWW.GIGISCLOSET.COM
A nice array of upscale brands such as Aubade and Lejaby, an abundance of lace plus a panty-of-the-month club.

WWW.GRAFFITIPINK.COM
Flirty line of colorful lingerie from Honeydew Intimates to State of Undress. Their own line of Graffiti Pink cotton undies is simple and fresh.

WWW.HERROOM.COM
Decent choice of brands and prices of lingerie basics from Bali to Chantelle. Easy to shop by color, as shades are listed under each piece on the main page.

WWW.HIPUNDIES.COM
Select but fun brands like Undiemoon and Mary Green. Comfy pj's galore.

WWW.NOWTHATSLINGERIE.COM
Amazing service for a Web site. Personal e-mails and offers of assistance are sent with each order. A well-curated selection including Arianne, Papillon Blanc, Triumph, and Change of Scandinavia Lingerie. Good prices, too.

WWW.PJSALVAGE.COM
Slip into oh-so-soft modal pajama sets in adorable and sassy prints from this website. The camis are so cute you'll want to show them off outside the bedroom. Prices are reasonable for these fresh styles.

WWW.VICTORIASSECRET.COM
Boobalicious padded bras to tiny panties. With "over 45 ways to get the cleavage you want," there's no secret as to what's going on here.

Sizing it Up

INTERNATIONAL SIZE CHARTS

*Refer to these charts when you're bra shopping overseas,
online or in a shop that carries European sizes.*

INTERNATIONAL BRA SIZE CHART

U.S.A.	EUROPE	FRANCE	U.K.	ITALY	AUSTRALIA
30	65	80	30		8
32	70	85	32	1	10
34	75	90	34	2	12
36	80	95	36	3	14
38	85	100	38	4	16
40	90	105	40	5	18

INTERNATIONAL PANTY SIZE CHART

U.S.A.	EUROPE	FRANCE	U.K.	ITALY	AUSTRALIA
XS	36 (1)	38 (1)	8	1	8
S	38 (2)	40 (2)	10	2	10
M	40 (3)	42 (3)	12	3	12
L	42 (4)	44 (4)	14	4	14
XL	44 (5)	46 (5)	16	5	16

Note: Some manufacturers may rely on a different system to determine bra or panty size. Be sure to verify if you have any questions when making an undergarment purchase. For example, "small" panties made by the French brand Simone Pérèle start at size 1, which is typically considered "extra small."

INTERNATIONAL CUP SIZE CHART

U.S.A.	EUROPE/FRANCE	U.K.	ITALY	AUSTRALIA
AA	AA	AA		
A	A	A	A	A
B	B	B	B	B
C	C	C	C	C
D	D	D	D	D
DD/E	E	DD	DD	DD
DDD/F	F	E	E	E
DDDD/G	G	F	F	F
DDDDD/H	H	FF		FF
DDDDDD/I		G		G
J		GG		GG
		H		H
		HH		HH
		J		J
		JJ		JJ
		K		

INDEX

An Intimate Guide

ABOUT THE AUTHORS

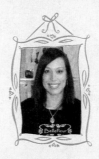

Jennifer Manuel Carroll is a lifelong lover of lingerie. With a background in sales and marketing, Carroll opened her popular shop, Bellefleur Lingerie Boutique, in the fashionable Fremont neighborhood of Seattle in 2002. Carroll is a savvy intimate-apparel expert: she can instantly guess a woman's bra size! She scouts for beautiful and provocative lingerie brands in her travels both locally and abroad. Her shop has been recognized by *Lucky Magazine* as one of the best places in the country to get a bra fitting.

When Carroll is not making over her clients' lingerie wardrobes, she enjoys traveling with her family (especially to France, land of luscious lingerie) and participating in local triathlons (she likes to keep her shapewear investment to a minimum). She currently resides in Seattle with her husband, Ryan, and two children. You can visit her shop online at www.bellefleurlingerie.com and reach her at jennifer@bellefleurlingerie.com.

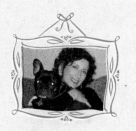

Kathy Schultz has written hundreds of articles on fashion, shopping, beauty, lifestyle and travel. She was the Seattle regional reporter for *Lucky Magazine*, the national shopping magazine, for seven years. Her work has also appeared in other periodicals, both national and local, within guidebooks and on Web sites.

Her lust for travel, fascination with other cultures and love of shopping have taken her to the flea markets of Paris, markets in the Provençal countryside, souks in Marrakech and, most recently, to the bazaars of India. She currently divides her time between Rajasthan, India, and Seattle, Washington. You can reach her at www.kathy-schultz.com.